Packed

Nutrient dense food for on the go lifestyles. Just because it may be eaten in the carpark while your kids are at activities or during your lunch break, does not mean it has to be tasteless and unhealthy!!

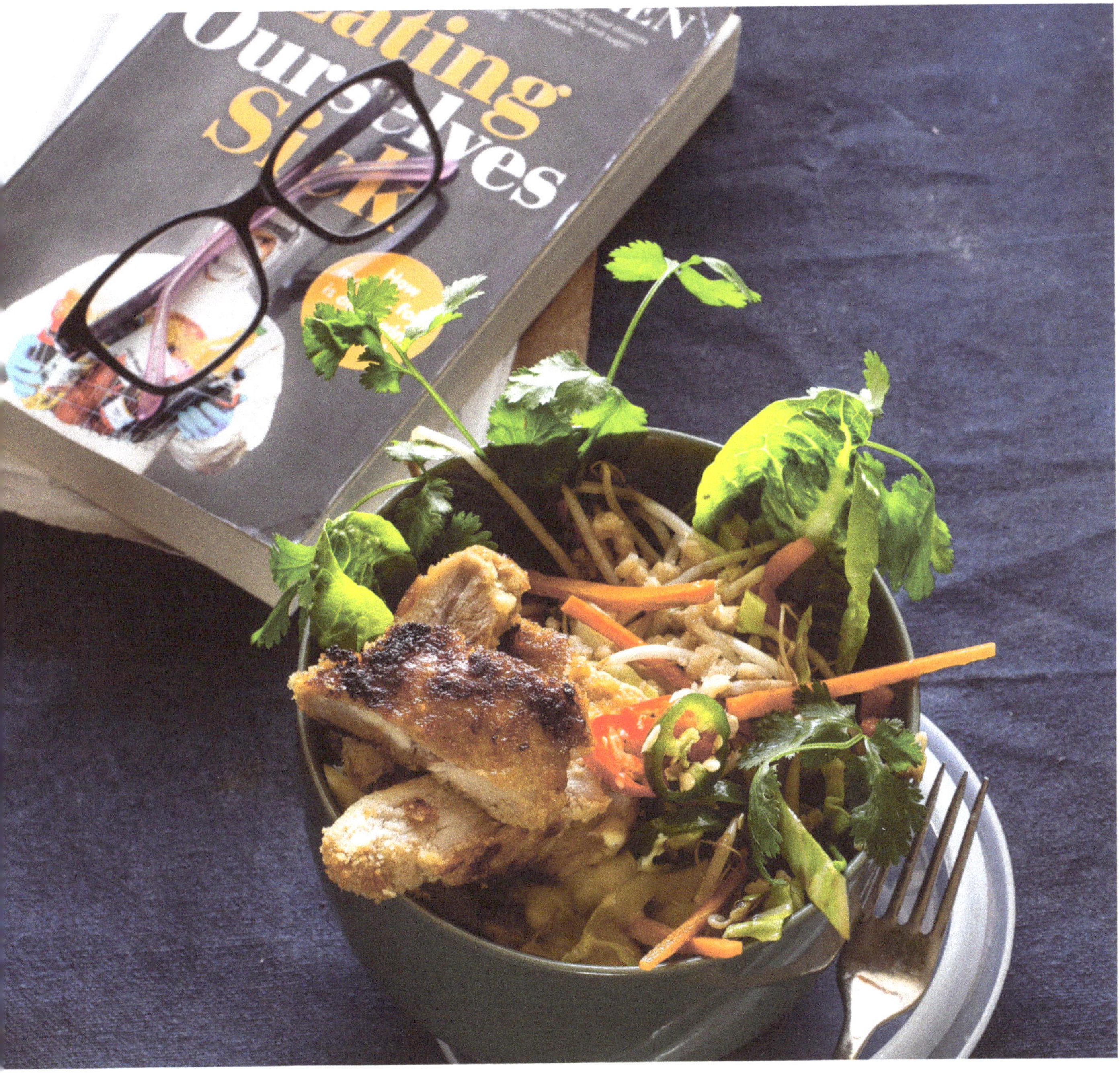

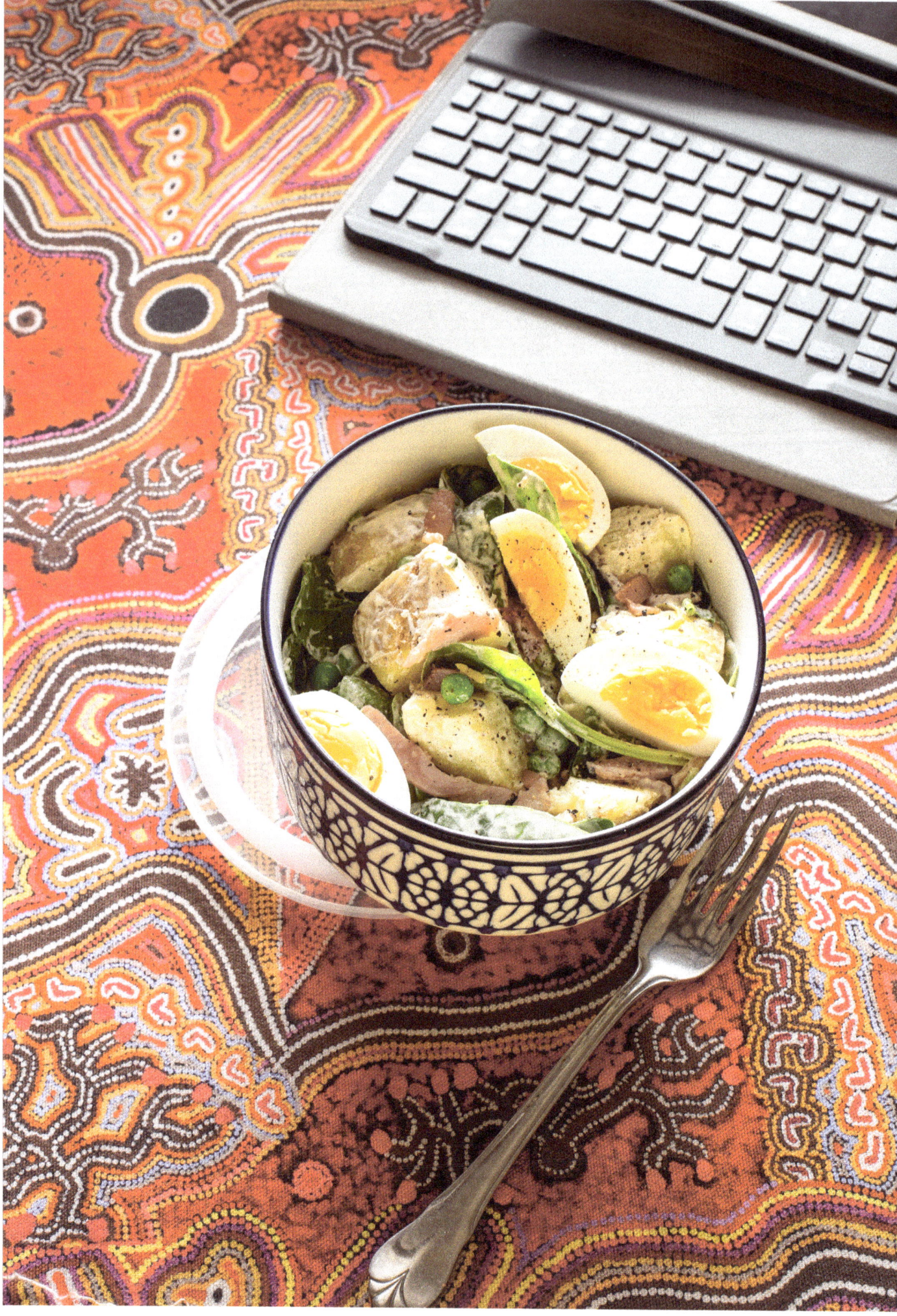

Introduction

You do not need to be chained to the kitchen sink all day every day to ensure you and your family are eating well, but be realistic, you need to be prepared to invest some time into organisation and preparation. The return on the investment is well worth it, your health. Improved energy levels from eating well will help you to achieve all your goals in life. Every single cell of your body needs good nutrition to grow and thrive, it is vitally important and should be a priority, don't you think? The modern 'quick and easy' approach to meal preparation is probably not helping, making most feel disappointed after spending an hour cooking and another hour cleaning up after the 'promised 5-minute meal'!

Whilst on summer holidays at our home in Eaglehawk Neck, our family meals are simple. Whatever fish is caught that day is served with potatoes and salads from the garden, topped with different dressings, chutneys and sauces. This way of eating is on repeat for a few weeks, with meat on the BBQ in between - it's our ideal way to eat. During the busy school terms I need to be more organised. The kids have activities 5 nights after school and most of Saturday. I might cook a roast lamb on a Sunday with enough roast veggies and meat for salads, sandwiches and wraps for the week. At the same time the roast is in the oven I'll have a chicken in the slow cooker making a delicious stock which will be the base for 3 or 4 meals, and a bolognaise or chilli con carne bubbling away in the thermocooker for another few meals. I will also have a slice in the oven and some wraps or scrolls on the go too. I like to use my freezer, so rather than cooking one batch of chilli con carne, I cook four. I keep the freezer well-stocked through the school terms so when I work all weekend at a Cooking Retreat or Indulgence Weekend at our business Little Norfolk Bay Events and Chalets, I still have a stack of healthy meal choices for the week. So an amazing weeknight meal might simply be created at 6am on a busy morning by heating the meat and whipping up a fresh salad to accompany it, not hard at all once organised! Once you start cooking this way you 'keep ahead' so there is always a variety of choices.

Wheat and other grains are cheap so are often used as fillers in takeaway and packaged products to bulk them out. I choose more nutrient dense meat, vegetables and fish, but I do enjoy bread more as a carrier for the good stuff, such as a home-made wraps filled with a full cup of salad and protein, or a slice of sourdough lathered with chicken liver pate. Home made pasta made with pretty much 50 percent egg and a good quality flour is quite high in protein in comparison to a supermarket brand packet of pasta that probably has cheap flour and additives to stick it together. You only need to think about how you feel after eating these foods to know which one is better. The home made version is satisfying and digests easily. However, we will use a packet pasta for a weeknight vegetable packed spaghetti bolognaise. There definitely are better choices of packet pasta and even some excellent vegetable options.

I try to not to get stuck in the school sandwich rut and when we do eat wheat, it is preferably a home-made sourdough for a slice of toast loaded with protein for breakfast, or a few tablespoons of flour amongst a kilo of zucchini in a slice. I have included wheat and dairy in this book, however, if you are cutting them out my recipes are easily modified. At times I have taken them out for periods (without making a song and dance just cut it out) which actually isn't at all that hard when starting with real food such as meat, eggs, fish, fruits and vegetables. I substitute brown rice or chickpea flour for wheat flour.

Like most things, cooking gets easier with practice. We should reflect, learn and improve. What might seem like an epic mission the first time, will soon become easier and your "normal" after several attempts. Home made wraps are a good example of this. It seems like a big task and the packet version is so much easier - but the flavour is amazing and is so worth the effort, let alone the unhealthy additives and preservatives that are in the packet varieties.

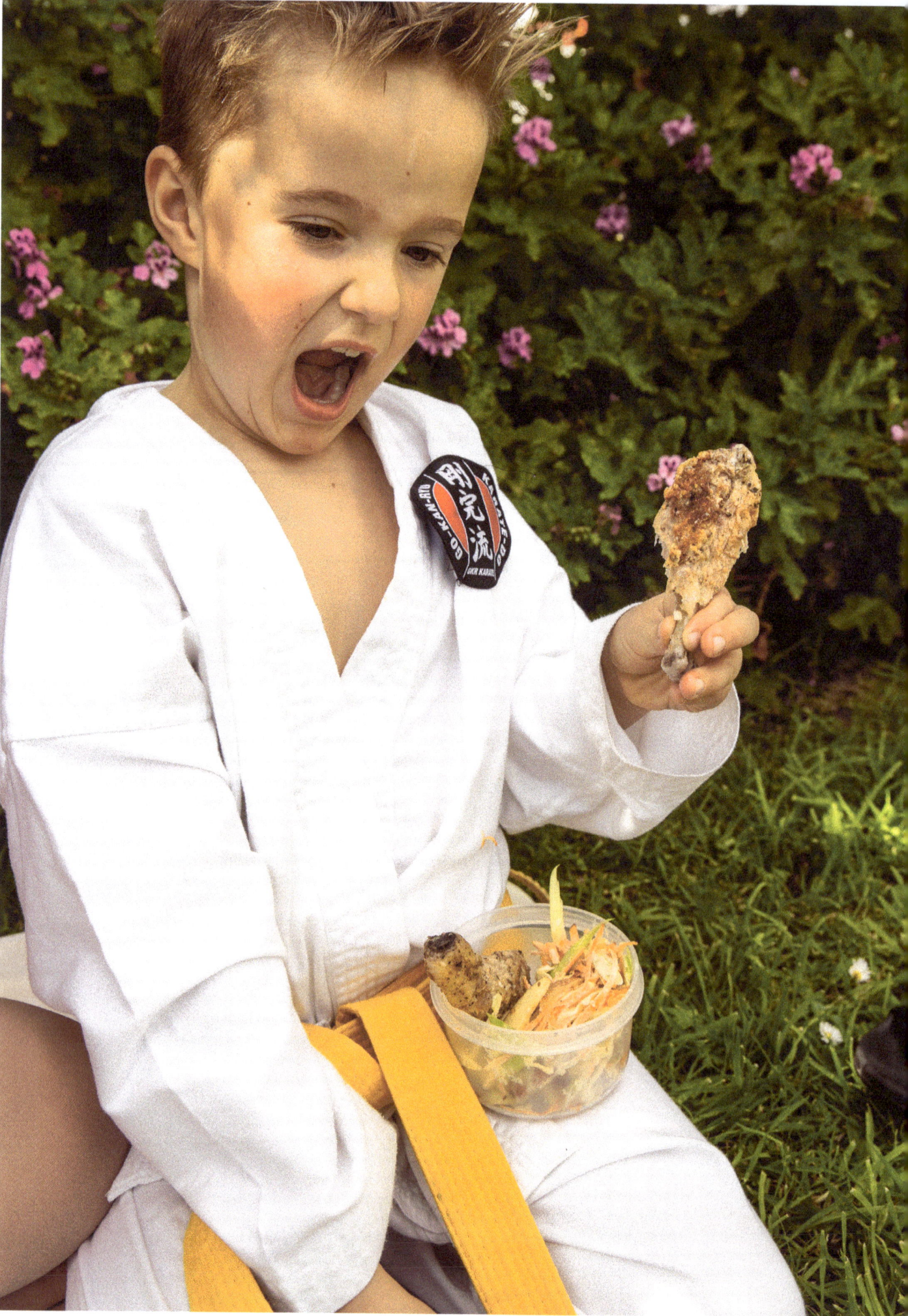

Always keep in mind that we are brainwashed by the commercial food industry into believing that cooking is time consuming and hard - and I am here to tell you it is not! When those people in the big offices that are creating their products are deciding their next marketing strategy, your health is not considered at all in their plans.

In our house the bulk of our meals made up from:

- good quality grass fed red meats
- fish & seafood
- extra virgin olive oil
- nuts
- approx. one kilo of vegetables and fruit a day per person
- and whatever else is need to make that all taste good, including a few serves of starchy carbs each day such as bread (preferably not white - choose better quality wholegrains or sourdough) rice, oats and pasta.
- I LOVE food and eating it - there's nothing better than to grow and cook a beautiful meal to enjoy. We have been brainwashed by the commercial food industry, that healthy is tasteless and this is simply not true. My kids would choose a home made burger or pizza over a fast food version any day! In fact, I feel sick now even walking past a greasy takeaway these days with the smell of the bad toxic vegetable oil. I feel revolting after a few slices of that cheap cheese and meat greasy pizza they are selling for $5 a pop!! (Seriously, what are they using on these to make them so cheaply?)

Eating is one of life's simple pleasures, so even if I am eating in the carpark at the kids dancing, I want it to be delicious and enjoyable, and for me to feel good and well nourished after eating it.

This book was created so I could share what I have learnt over many years of being a chef, and most recently being a busy mum of three very active children. We have a very full life - we live on the Tasman Peninsula, and my children attend a school in Hobart. For most of the past 10 years I commuted daily with the children to take them to school. I also take them to their many activities outside of school such as dancing, karate, football, cricket, swimming, art classes, acting classes and more. My husband is often away for work for long periods so I had to do this by myself a majority of the time. I run a busy accommodation and cooking workshop retreat on the Tasman Peninsula and I am a freelance photographer and foodstylist.

But I never allowed this to be an excuse to not find time to cook nutritious meals. Beside the fact that it would cost a fortune to feed my family on takeaways - the cost on their health was just something I am not willing to compromise on. For women it is not anti-feminist to cook and spend time in the kitchen and choose to be healthy, we can have a career and cook meals too -with every family member taking on some responsibilities in the kitchen and towards thier own good health!

Happy cooking,

Eloise Emmett

Why?

So why bother putting all that effort in cooking your food?

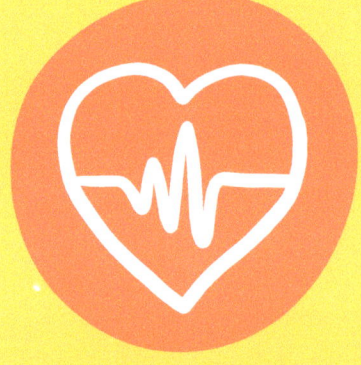

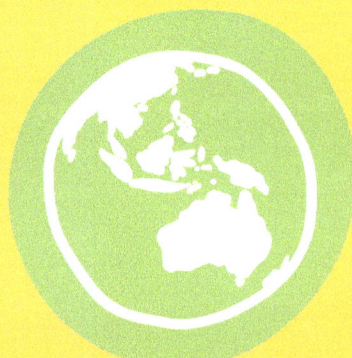

Cost for your wallet

Cost for your health

Cost for the planet

Cooking your food is always the most economical choice. I prefer to spend my money on the fun activities my kids do that keep them active, which then circles back to them having "exercise" that they enjoy. Some people believe that takeaway food is cheap, but for a meal to feed my family at a takeaway shop, it costs $60-$120 and I can buy a lot of veggies and meat with that! Not to mention that it has little nutritional value so is just a waste.

There are endless amounts of research you can find on the effects of not eating well. We know it contributes to obesity, heart disease, depression, anxiety and more. You can find the information easily yourself. It is pretty confronting to sadly see that pharmaceutical companies currently define lifestyle illnesses as "growth industries" worth investing in.

Did you know that 20% of food that is purchased will never be eaten? It is just thrown away. All that time, energy and resources that went into making that food - all gone. 60% of the Australian diet is discretionary foods, foods that provide little or no nutrition or are even health negative. Isn't that just a ridiculous waste too? Just think of your own fridge and pantry - how much goes to waste? With better organisation with your meals, not only will your health benefit, but so will the planet.

Check out the breakdown of this delicious meal that uses top quality ingredients and is full of nutrition. You can find the recipe on page 122

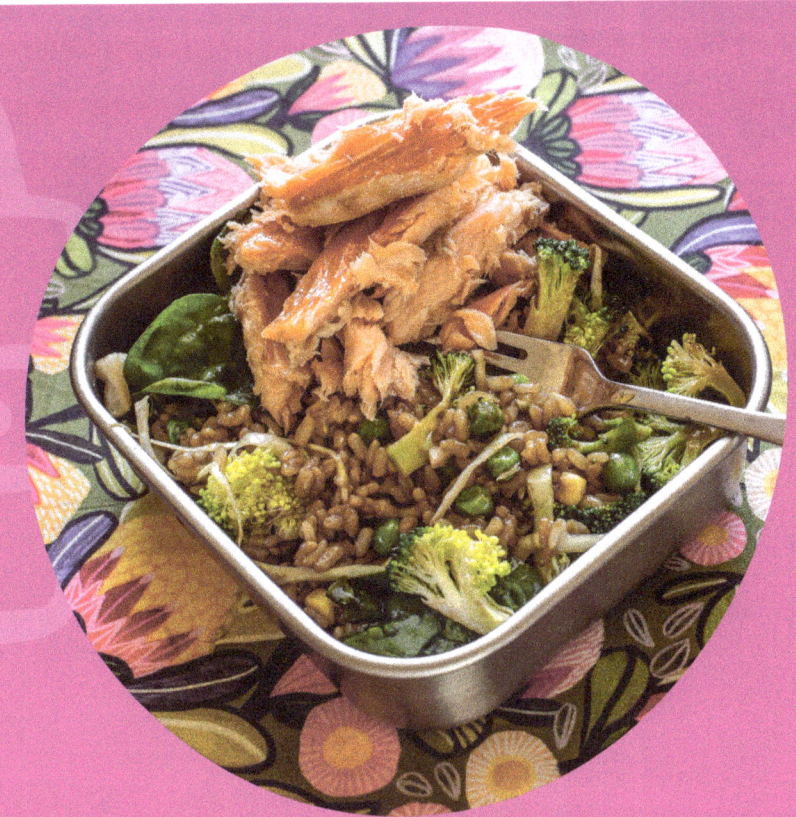

Honey Soy Brown Rice Salad with Tassal Hot Smoked Salmon

I have worked out the cost of this gorgeous salmon salad that makes about five serves and is one of my favourite cold packed meals. Living in Tassie I am lucky enough to be able to pick up the economical salmon offcuts from the Salmon Shop Salamanca, so I always have them in the freezer. The salmon shop has a truck that we can buy from in regional Tasmanian areas. I also use Tassal Cooked Tassie Salmon (Naturally Smoked), even when this recipe is made with the premium product the cost per serve is still way more economical than a take away.

3 tablespoons (60 ml) extra virgin olive oil ($30 /litre)	$1.80
2 tables spoon white vinegar ($2 /litre)	$0.08
1 tablespoon (20 ml) honey ($28/kilo)	$0.56
1 tablespoon soy (20 ml) ($4/500 ml)	$0.16
¼ teaspoon sea salt	$0.05
¼ teaspoon pepper	$0.05
1.5 cups brown ($5/2 kilo)	$0.75
1 cup peas ($4/kilo)	$.80
1 cup corn ($5/kilo)	$1.00
tin white beans ($ 2/can)	$2.00
small head broccoli ($4 kilo)	$0.80
1 cup cabbage ($4/kilo)	$0.60
2 cups spinach leaves ($5 bag)	$2.50
500 grams Tassal hot smoked salmon pieces	$7.50
or 500 grams Tassal Cooked Tasssie Salmon (naturally smoked)	
TOTAL COST	$18.65
Per Serve (5 in total)	$3.73

$3.73 per serve!
What could you buy for less than $4 in a takeaway store? A few greasy chips? 2 potato cakes?

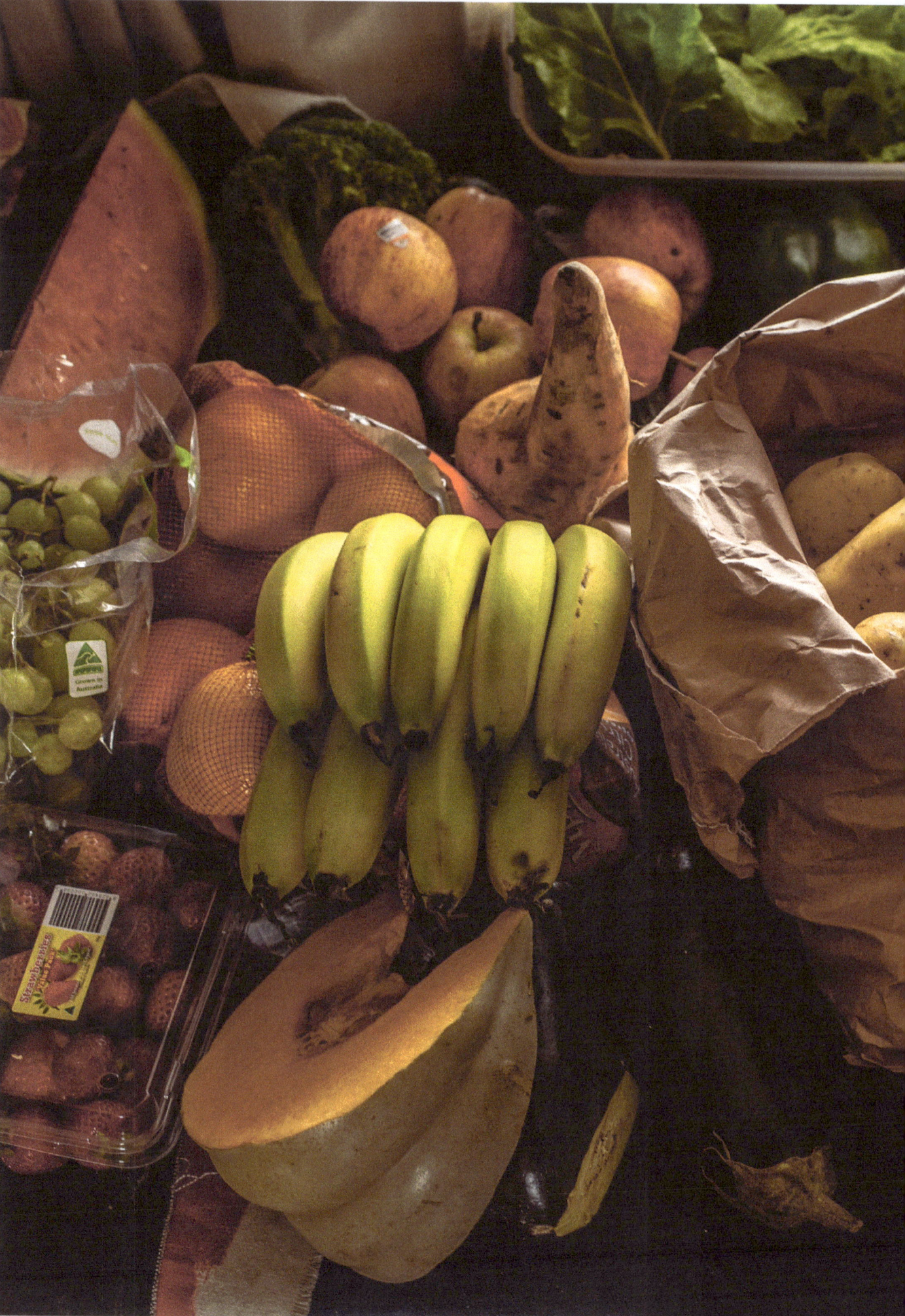

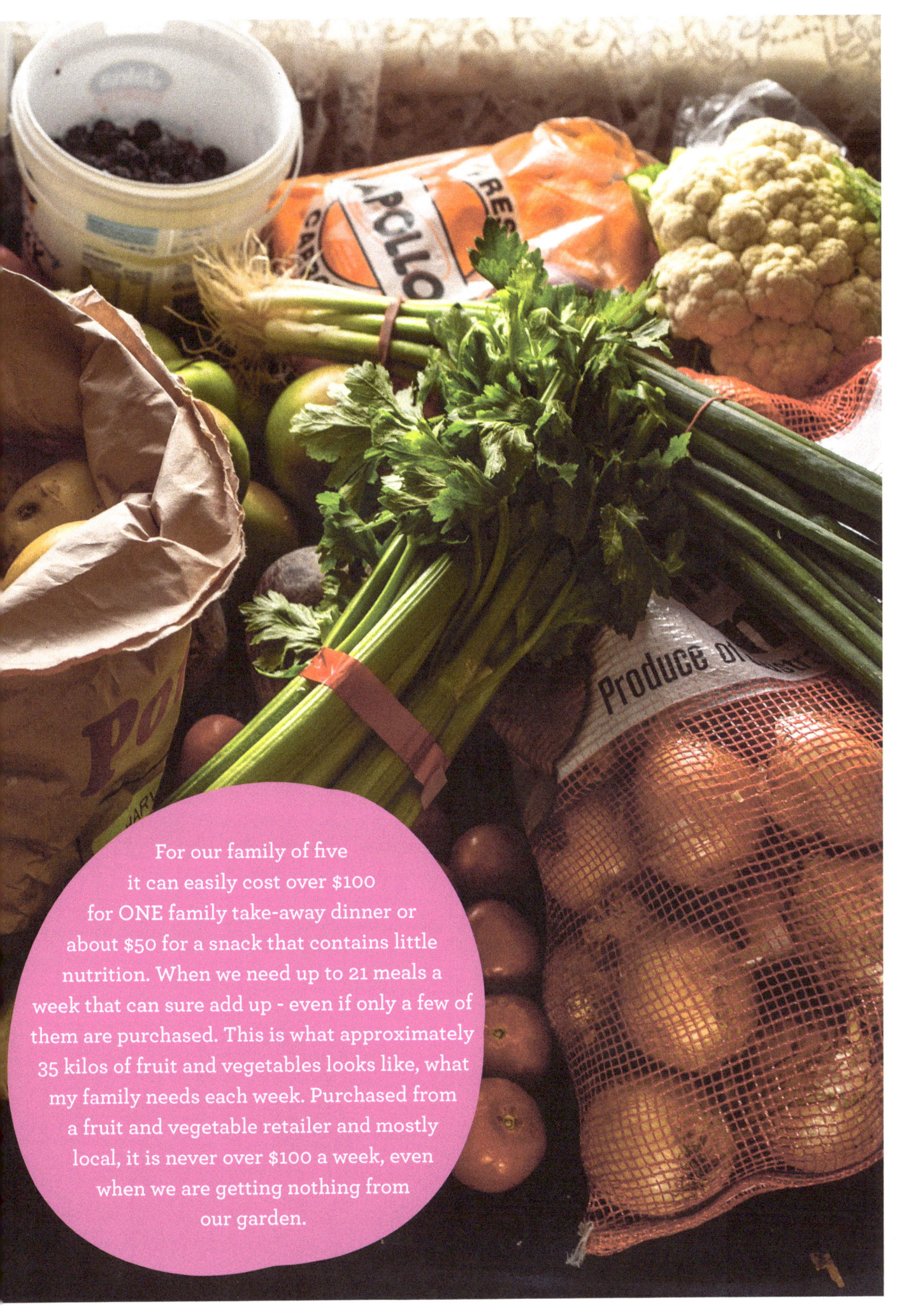

For our family of five it can easily cost over $100 for ONE family take-away dinner or about $50 for a snack that contains little nutrition. When we need up to 21 meals a week that can sure add up - even if only a few of them are purchased. This is what approximately 35 kilos of fruit and vegetables looks like, what my family needs each week. Purchased from a fruit and vegetable retailer and mostly local, it is never over $100 a week, even when we are getting nothing from our garden.

Cost for your health

DEFINITION OF HEALTHY

Unfortunately we have "diet culture" to mess with our heads and it gets hard to figure out what is actually healthy when there are isles of fat, sugar and salt filled empty calorie food like substances filling supermarkets labeled "healthy" or "natural". It is so confusing as to what is actually healthy. Disgustingly, pharmaceutical companies lied about the BMI in the 80s and convinced everyone that our sole life purpose was to lose weight to fit into their never achievable narrow margin of acceptable. And to help us, they then invented the multi-billion dollar a year industry of dumb weight loss programs and products!

Believe me, like most women my age born in that era, I've tried all those stupid diets and have been a lot thinner, but I can clearly see now my thinest was NOT my healthiest! Choosing real whole foods and focusing on my gut health seem the easiest way for me to be my best. With a goal of high energy levels and a good mood so I can parent to the best of my ability rather then be small, low in energy and grumpy as hell!

YOUR ENERGY

I have found over the years a healthy diet involves being organised as I need good food in the fridge and pantry to easily make nutrient dense meals for energy. It's too easy being a parent to put your own needs last and it's easy to slip into bad habits that start a cycle of low energy - can't be bothered cooking, not sleeping well, extra alcohol and caffeine, bloating and constipation etc. etc. If the revolting greasy foods are looking appetising, there is a problem - you are starving, and it really does form a cycle. Doing the work and getting in good habits, prioritising good sleep, eliminating or cutting down alcohol, prioritising exercise that you enjoy and cooking and eating well, gets easy when you are doing it all. Most importantly I want to be a good example for my kids so they learn to cook and feed themselves well.

YOUR GUT MICROBIOME

For great gut health, I try to eat 30 different plants each week. I am not trying to say I am an expert or qualified as such in this area, this is not medical advice BUT I am pretty obsessed with my gut microbiome and there is overwhelming amount of research to show that it is the basis of good health and is so important for mental health. What frustrates me the most is when the commercial food industry just loves to jump on fads, and gut health is it's latest. Don't be fooled - you don't need their fancy and expensive products. If you are cooking your food from real ingredients and following the basics of the Mediterranean style diet of approximately a kilo of fruit and vegetables a day, you are probably doing a pretty good job already. Including meals like a weekly roast meal with all the vegetables, homemade baked beans for breakfast and salads for lunches, then you probably already have a pretty healthy gut! You certainly don't need to be buying packets labelled "good for your gut" or pre or probiotic. For example expensive packets of cereals that are labelled prebiotic when it is just the everyday oats in the box that contain the prebiotics - tricky and sneaky marketing!!.

This is what I have learnt and do:

- eat a at least 30 different plants a week
- include prebiotics found in foods like oats, onions, garlic and other veggies and fruits - easy when you are cooking most of your meals
- eat something fermented each day for probiotics such as olives (naturally fermented), fermented mustards, kimchi, sauerkraut, kombucha or kefir
- drink plenty of pure water
- move (find ways to exercise you enjoy)
- sleep well
- eliminate or cut down food additives and preservatives and nasty oils, which is not at all hard to do when starting with vegetables and meat. Surely our bodies struggle to process that stuff, it must have an effect somewhere!
- cut down or out coffee and alcohol

I don't have to do a 4 year degree in dietetics to know that a homemade version, as well as being insanely delicious, made from top quality grass fed meat, loads of fresh salad and vegetables, and only good oil, is so much better for you. You only need to judge how you feel after eating them. And way more economical too!

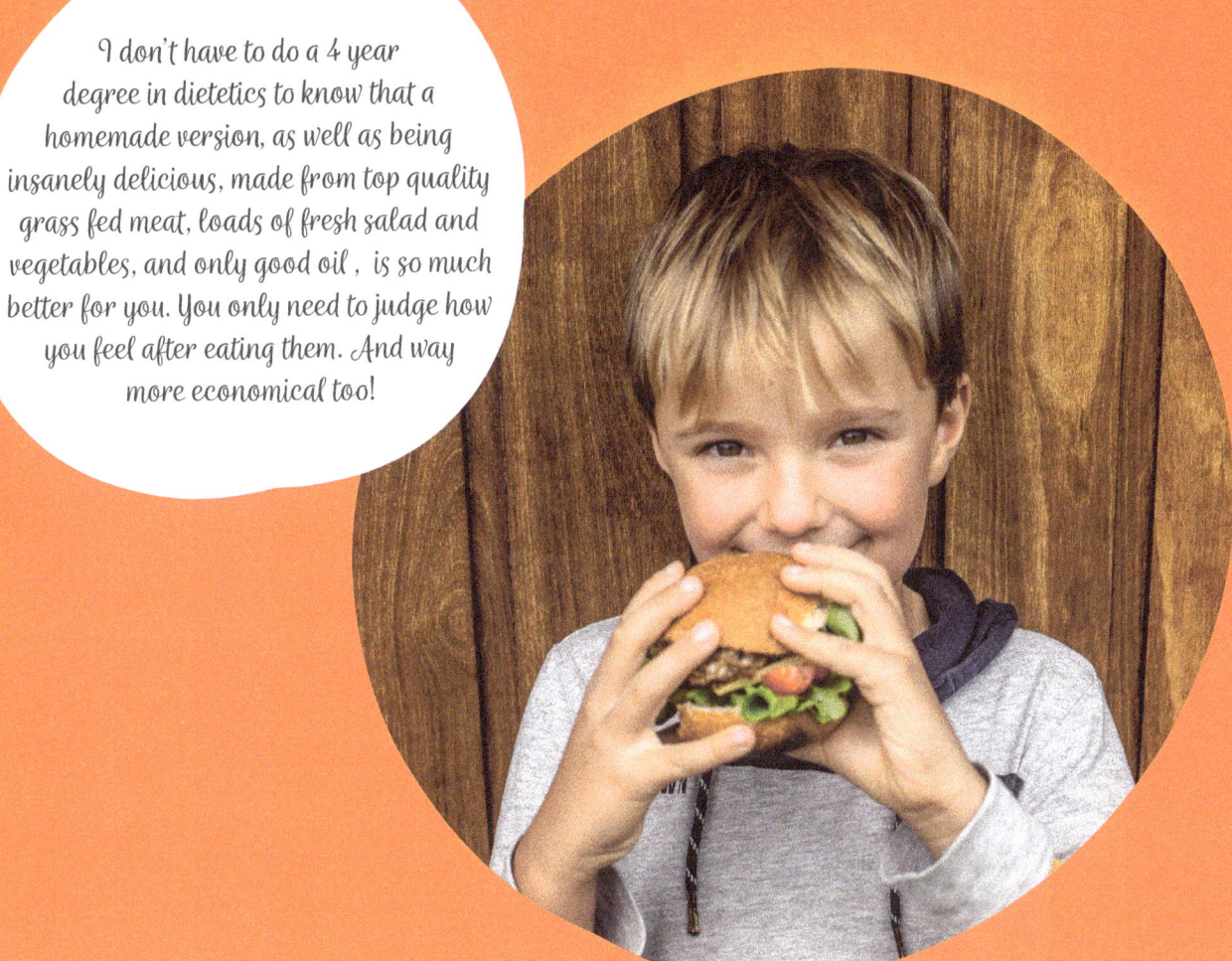

YOU ARE WHAT YOU EAT, AND DO, AND THINK

There is endless amounts of research you can find on the effects of not eating well. We know a bad diet contributes to obesity, heart disease, depression, anxiety, even cancers and more. Often we are told that these illnesses are passed down in our genes, and there's not a whole lot we can do to prevent them. The standard treatment is usually medicine and often there isn't a cure. While medication can be great, it can also start a rollercoaster of side effects, more medication to treat side effects, and no cure, just a management of symptoms. So prevention or finding the root cause would be far better, don't you think? Yes, I'm not a doctor and you should always consult your trusted doctor for health advice, but make sure you find one that is more interested in prevention and finding out the root cause of your illness. I knew I found myself a great doctor when she was interested in what I was eating, my sleep patterns and my stress levels.

Your genes play an important role in your health, but so do your behaviors and environment, such as what you eat and how physically active you are. Look up the study of epigenetics. It's really quite fascinating!

To put epigenetics in simple terms, our genes respond to what we put in our environment - the air we breathe, the food we consume, the exercise we do and our thought patterns. So, if you think you are unhealthy and there is nothing you can do as you have bad genes – that doesn't seem to be the case. Instead of thinking of diseases as just hereditary, perhaps there are also hereditary habits that get passed down generation to generation? Interesting isn't it?

It is hard to accept that you may have contributed to your own disease or your child's illness, but you only know what you know, when you know it and we are all just trying to do our best. But when we know better we can do better, it is never too late to change and break the cycle!

Cost for the planet

WASTE

Let's talk about the waste of eating food that is providing no nutritional value. The average Australian diet is made up of 60 percent discretionary foods, food that provides little or no nutrition value - some even health negative. 60 percent of all food produced is NOT NEEDED which is completely ridiculous! This is before we worry about the 20 percent of food purchased that's tossed in the bin. The impact on the environment and people's health is insane. When I see figures like this I can't believe our governments don't step in and do something. So, if you are worried about the environment then cooking and only (or mostly) eating nutritious foods is a good start anyway!

As fantastic as it is to have so much choice, sometimes we need get back to eating what you need to, rather than what you feel like. Looking at the last vegetables at the bottom of the crisper and turning them into a yummy soup rather than throwing them out is a good place to start. Because most of us buy our fruit and vegetables from stores, sometimes we don't realise how hard it really is to grow them. If you've ever grown your own fruit and vegetables, you are much less inclined to waste any of them! Always cook what needs to be used first and try really hard not to throw nothing away.

Perhaps have a few meals a week that are "what needs to be eaten" and educate your kids too and make it a normal part of your week. For example, Thursday dinner may be eating "whatever is in the fridge night", not a planned meal as such. One person may have left over lamb and salad, another the leftover spaghetti bolognaise and another the leftover soup and eggs on toast. The leftover carrot and celery sticks from the lunchbox can go in the stock. And if there is food left in the kids lunchboxes offer them that after school before anything else. You don't need to cook a meal every night of the week - it is OK to eat leftovers and it gives you a night off!

PLASTICS

Can you imagine if everyone stopped eating packet food - what a huge reduction in the need for plastics! When you cut out packaged food - you are not only helping to heal your own body, you are helping to minimise the use of plastics and packaging.

It is estimated that 300 million tons of plastic is produced every year, and half of this plastic is used just once and then disposed.

It is estimated that 150 million metric tons of plastic circulate the world's oceans. It is estimated that by 2050 there will be more plastic in the oceans than fish.

By cooking more of your food from scratch from whole foods you will heal yourself and the environment!

SNACK CULTURE

I get asked all the time for healthy snack recipes. This is another fad that has been pushed onto us by the commercial food industry.

I find if I eat 2-3 good meals a day with adequate protein, all I need for a snack is some fruit and vegetables to munch on.

Kids might need a snack after school or in the lunchbox on days when they are off to a few hours of exercise. Air popped popcorn drizzled with extra virgin olive oil and sea salt, nuts, cheese are good simple choices. I do have a few recipes in this book for after school and lunch box items but in general, I think our obsession with "healthy snacks" is actually extremely unhealthy and is probably filling us up before mealtime and adding extra energy we may not need.

It drove me crazy when my kids were young when playgroup facilitators would STOP the kids happily playing (moving and exercising) for a snack break and all the party food wrapped in plastic would come out of the lunchboxes! Kids will eat when they are hungry.

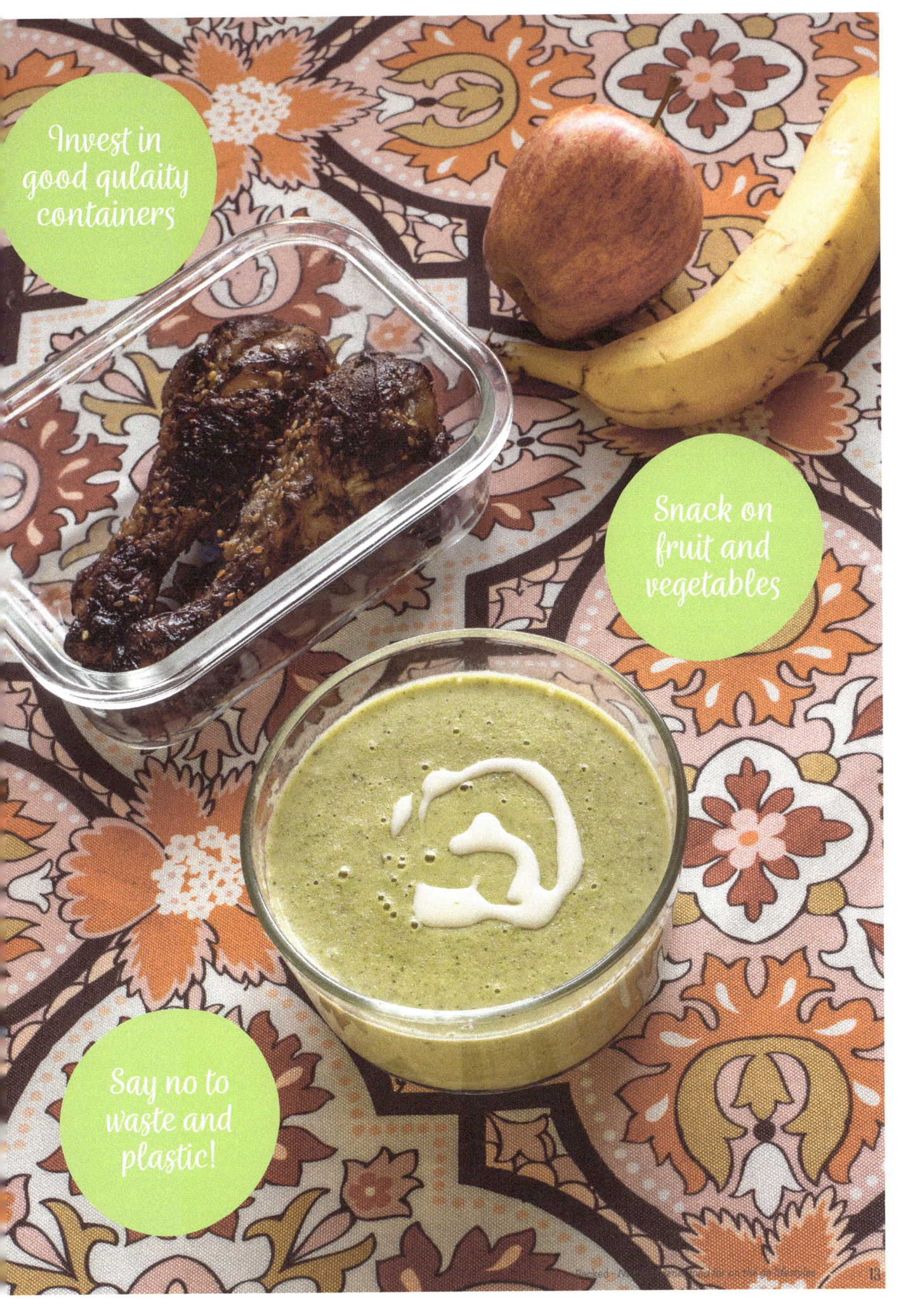

How?

So how do we do it?

EQUIPMENT

I would have to recommended one really good sharp cook's knife, it is really worth the investment. I love my thermocooker as you can see I use it for so many of my recipes. The thermocooker, as well as being a great blender, is really a pot that stirs itself while cooking, so super handy for busy parents. It is worth investing in some really good containers to pack hot and cold foods. If you're on a budget, perhaps check out the op shops. I choose to spend my money on good things for my kitchen that make cooking that little bit easier and enjoyable. As we have established, its pretty important for our health, unlike big TVs or couches that other people may choose to spend their money on, that are effectively health negative.

KIDS IN THE KITCHEN

Get the kids in the kitchen when they are young to help with the basics. It may be really annoying and take longer, but persevere, as they get older they will become handy little helpers. I would say by 7 years old they should be able to pack their own lunch and by 10 years old, cook a basic dinner.

Of course I would not allow young children in the kitchen when there is hot fat bubbling away for deep frying, and there does need to be care taken around hot and sharp objects.

When doing Facebook live cooking demonstrations, I have had people freak out when Oscar was young playing with a grater. Seriously, what's the risk? A grated finger! What's the risk of NOT teaching them to cook and eat well? Obesity, heart disease, depression?...

FUSSY EATERS

They need to get over it. If ultra-processed food like substances were not available and only real food was, your kids would eat it. As a human species we want to survive. Don't offer the junk, be prepared to say no a lot to the requests to all the ultra-processed food like substance forced in their faces everywhere, even at sports! Yes, this is hard and frustrating walking into the pool for swimming lessons you need to walk past the fridges of ice-creams and lollies, it really annoys me. Why the government does nothing when the rates of lifestyle created diseases are rising and probably filling up the health system?

But the more people there are who are feeding their kids real food, the easier it is for us, as this becomes the normal! I keep the good food in the house and the ultra processed foods out.

FEEDING KIDS

I work on the recommended principle that it is my (or with my husband, our) job to provide the food, and it is our children's job to decide what and how much they eat. I do try to include food they love as much as I can but if they don't like it and do not eat it then they don't get offered anything else. They can grab a vegetable from the fridge and eat that, but they will have to wait for the next meal. As such, I do not have any overly fussy eaters in my household. People say I am lucky my children are not fussy - but it has nothing to do with luck. Don't cater to fussy eaters and you wont have any!

I strongly believe that part of the brainwashing by food marketing has created a belief that kids don't eat enough

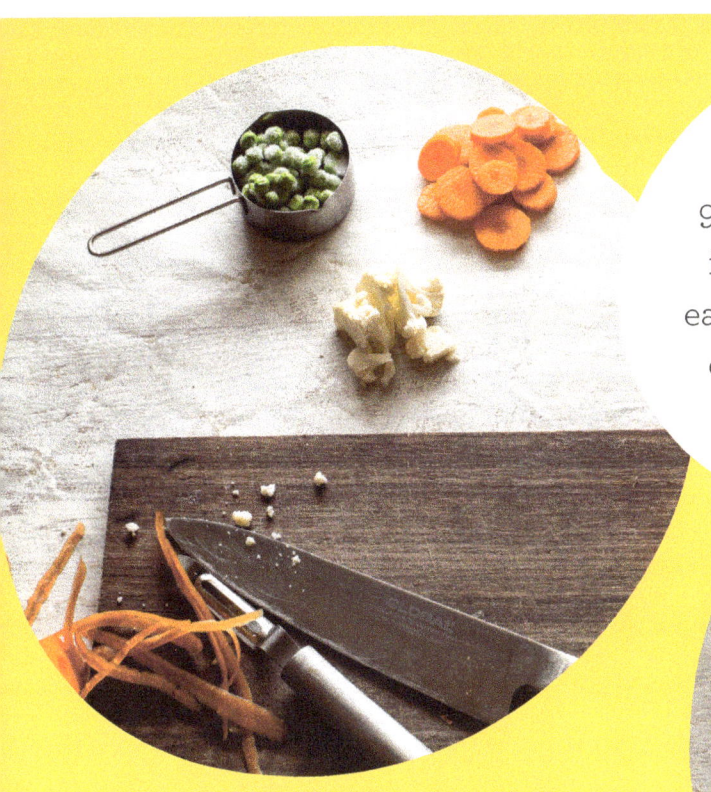

2.5 serves of vegetables

> Did you know that 96 percent of people in Tasmania do not eat enough vegetables each day. Why not? It is so easy!

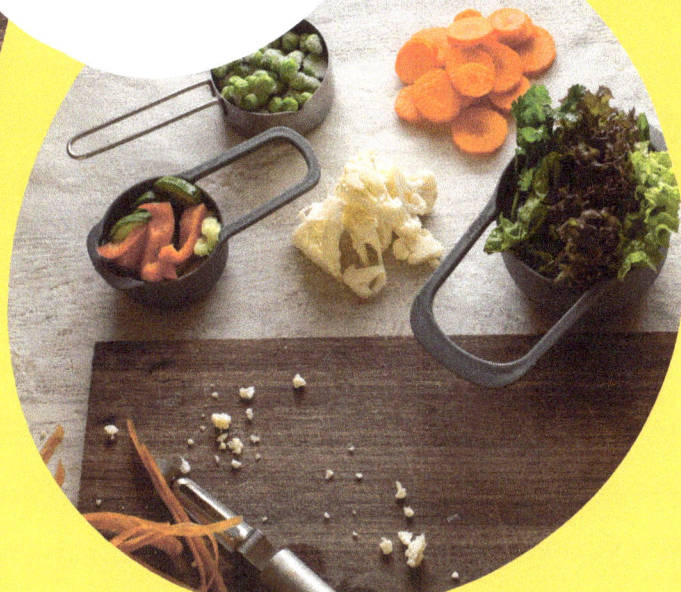

5 serves of vegetables

when they are young. But when they are young kids don't need to eat a lot - people are imagining piles of vegetables they need to eat. It is recommended and 2-3 year old eats 2.5 serves of veggies each day, one serve is about 75 grams or 1/2 cup veggies, one cup leafy greens it is really not a lot!! They want us to buy their ultra processed crap that contains a minute portion of nutrients and probably damaging their developing taste buds to a preference for the strategically concocted highly palatable sweet stuff. Some of the products are laughable 'contains spinach' on the packet may equate to one gram of spinach!

GET YOUR SERVE

Adults following the Mediterranean style diet will eat approximately one kilo of fruit and vegetables per person per day. While that sounds like a lot, one apple can weigh 150 grams, so it's not a huge amount really. One tomato with breakie, one apple as a snack, a cup of salad at lunch in a wrap, orange as a snack and veggies with dinner and it is easy done!! But do not listen to me, I am just a chef who only finished grade 10, listen to your body! How do you feel after eating this way?

I find it important to have some kind of plan for the week so I make sure I end up eating enough veggies each day. To make it go down easier, I use beautiful oils and vinegars and other condiments plus herbs and spices. A simple lunch would be leftover roast lamb plus balsamic, plus robust extra virgin olive oil, a few sweet and sour pickles and garlicky tzatziki - a simple and delicious meal.

Have the good ingredients on hand and treat yourself with fancy expensive ones sometimes, it is your health after all!

KITCHEN SKILLS

The recipes in my books are all very well tested however our oven temperatures will be different my 180°C oven will be slightly different than any other oven. Our scales will all be a bit different, probably even our cup and spoon measures. The fat content of the meat and seafood we use will be different. The size or thickness of the meat or fish will differ. The flours may be dryer so may need more moisture and the fruits and veggies will be of different sizes and water and sugar content. All of these things will affect the end result with cooking times. You need to learn to cook, you need to get a feel for it and understand it, I can guide you but I can not do it for you! If something goes wrong have a think about it and do it better the next time. Cooking a beautiful meal is one of life's simple pleasures why not enjoy it and feel great when you cook and enjoy something delicious. Practice and learn from it.

FOOD SAFETY

Some people worry about the food safety of reheating foods and then packing them to keep hot but the risks really are miniscule and if they are going to happen could happen at home anyway. To the best of my knowledge, I have never had or given anyone food poisoning in my life of home and commercial cooking. People can be scared of seafood and believe it is an allergen when hardly anyone is actually allergic to it. Eggs and chicken will contain salmonella but it is something like 1 in 20,000 and when stored and cooked properly is a non issue anyway.

I still have a giggle with my mum about some of her old fashioned ways when we were young, like leaving a big pot of pea and ham soup on the stove for days and it "just needs a good boil" each day to kill and germs. Or the old-fashioned Christmas spreads we enjoyed with ham and the

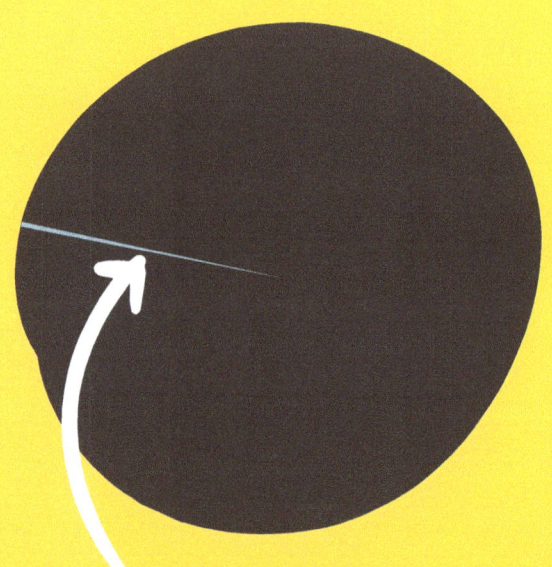

Chance of getting sick from cooking and eating real food

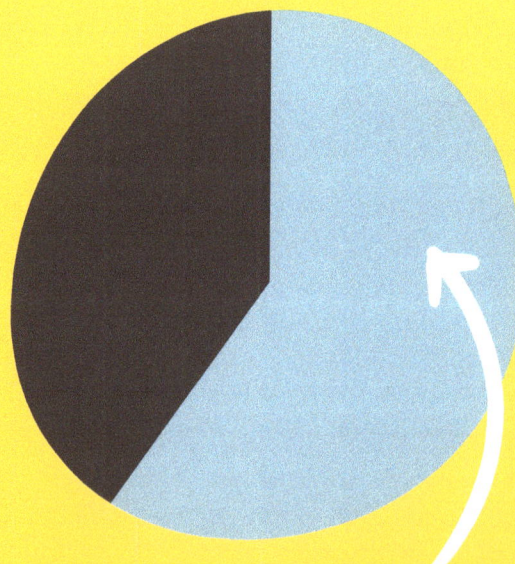

Chance of developing a lifestyle disease from ultra-processed food

Food poisoning affects 4 million people in Australia each year, it is a serious for certain people, but it is likely not from fresh well handled food cooked with care!!

works, left out for hours. It was only the generation before my mum that stored meat in a cupboard.

I strongly believe my childhood outside and at Bruny Island in the mud coupled with mums questionable food storage methods, is why I never really get sick now. This has actually contributed to good gut health. I remember times in my earlier working days gastro would be going around different workplaces and me just picking up a heap of extra shifts as everyone else was off work sick!

I would probably suggest that the food poisoning/food hygiene risks are blown out of proportion by the big food industries as part of their marketing (or should we call it brain washing). People can be a bit scared of real food like eggs, chicken, fish and even meat for food safety reasons. Wallaby, kangaroo and octopus, which is some of our first nations diet and most natural food can be considered gross, yet eating chemical laden food from plastic is OK? It is really nuts when you think about it! The chemically made factory packet food is even served in hospitals! Margarine for example is made from dirty oil that goes through 22 different chemical processes to end up in that tub! Extra virgin olive oil is fresh squeezed juice from the olive, full of amazing antioxidants that run around your body killing off the baddies (that's how I explain it to my kids!) Butter is from milk from the cow. Just have a little think about what you are eating.

There is a such low chance of food poisoning eating real food, and we now know the chemical laden processed food is contributing to 60 percent of the population having a lifestyle disease! Don't believe what big food tells you!

TIPS FOR FOOD SAFETY

- Make sure your fridge temperatures are checked often as bacteria will grow in the right conditions if it is running too warm or the seals are damaged.

- Keep ice blocks in the freezer all the time to keep your food cool when packing. and carting.

- Make sure your chicken and poultry is cooked through.

- Make sure you trust your retailer and the food is fresh when purchased. We get our grass fed beef direct from the farm and the rest of our meat from butchers who have pride in what they are doing. When we buy seafood it's from a seafood wholesaler or retailer that we trust.

- Try to cool food that needs to be cooled as quickly as possible.

- Reheat to a temperature that will kill the germs.

- Keep your workspaces and tools clean and wash dishcloths at least every day. I am not a fan of chemical kitchen sprays in the home kitchen. I use a vinegar & bicarb spray with a few drops of Port Arthur Lavender oil in it, in the kitchen. Vinegar's cleaning capabilities are really interesting if you have not looked into it.

- Wash up in very hot soapy water and rinse well, air dry where you can.

- Have some good containers for the fridge (this helps with waste too).

- Stack the fridge with meat, fish and chicken at the bottom, so if they do spill they will not drip on fresh foods that will not be cooked.

- Importantly, rotate your food, even flours and dry goods and nuts as they are a fresh product. Use the old first and keep a good eye on what you are buying so you use it up.

- Consume in the order needed, for example, if you do one big shop, the fish or chicken is used before the beef, which will keep longer.

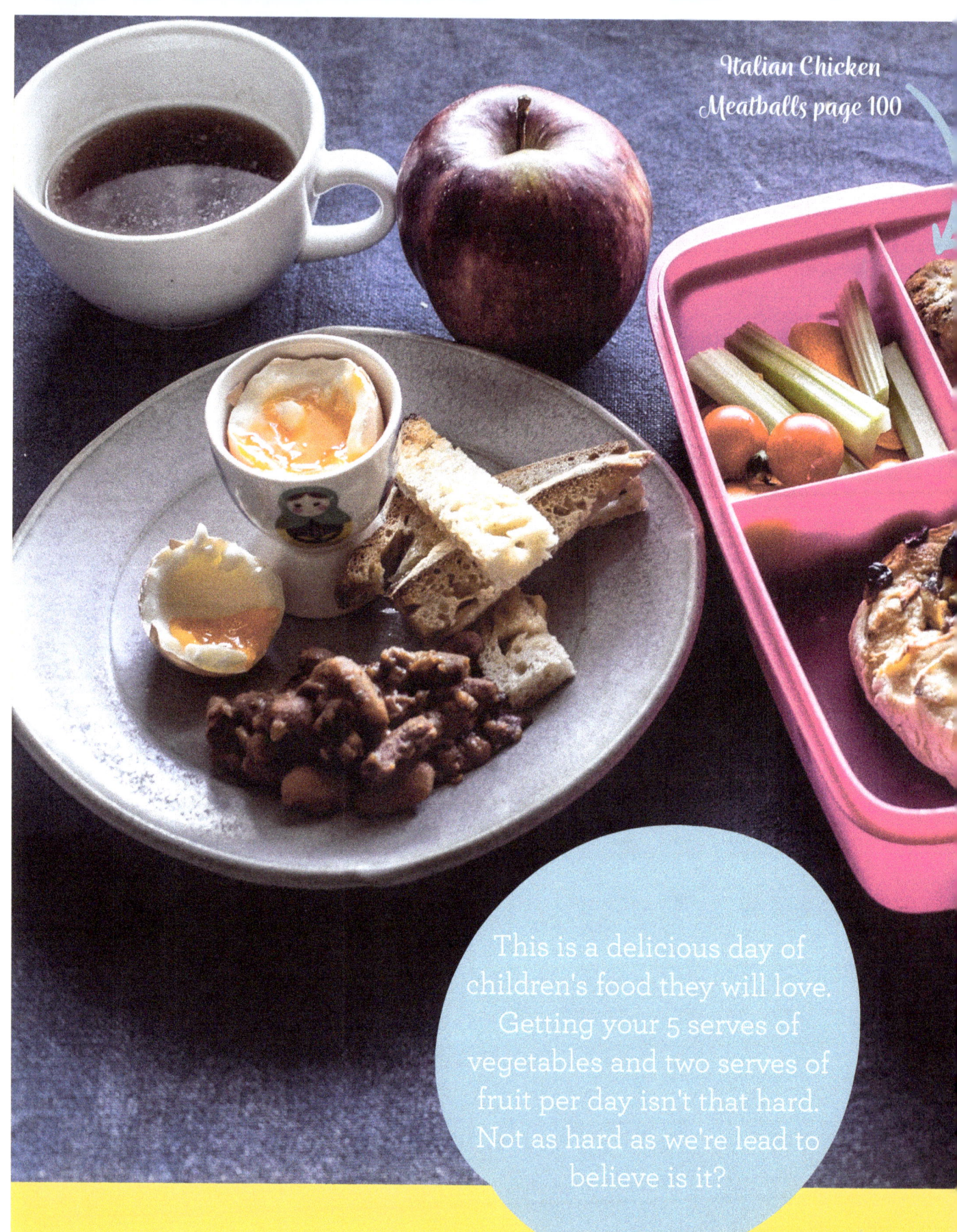

Italian Chicken Meatballs page 100

This is a delicious day of children's food they will love. Getting your 5 serves of vegetables and two serves of fruit per day isn't that hard. Not as hard as we're lead to believe is it?

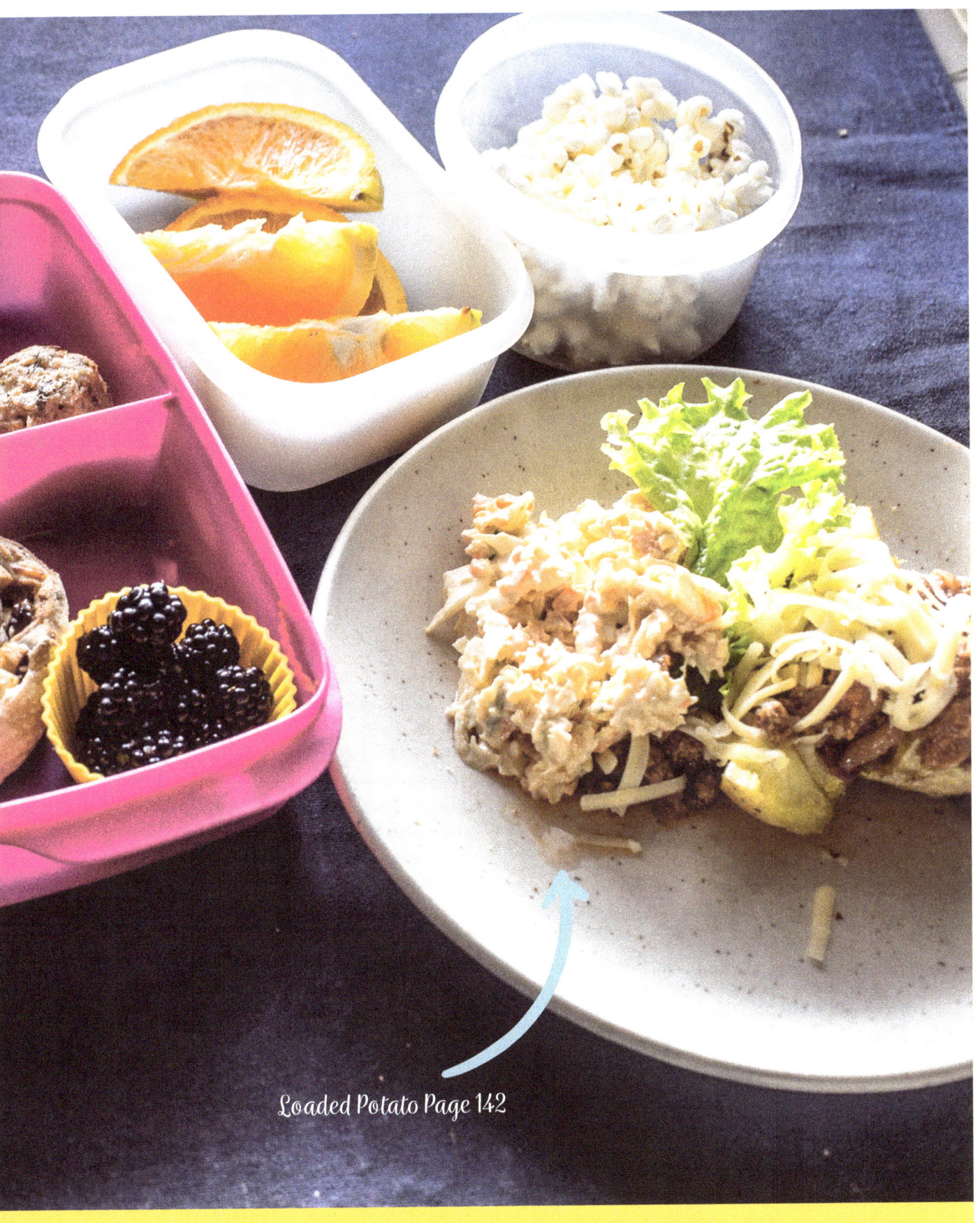

Loaded Potato Page 142

It takes about 5 minutes to make a batch of scrolls, 3 minutes to whip up a bowl of coleslaw, 10 minutes to put on a bolognaise, 5 minutes to put baked beans in the slow-cooker, 3 minutes to make the chicken balls. With plenty of food now prepared, there is less time needed on other days. Time to make all this? One TV show? A scroll through social media? It is not hard or time consuming!

Planning

Maybe it is because I had those angry Chefs in my ear during my apprenticeship constantly talking about the "6 Ps" for years, but investing some time into planning will help you out a lot! Meal planning does not have to be every veggie you are eating that week chopped up into little containers (and good for you if that's the way to choose to do it!) but having a rough idea of what you will be eating so you know you will be eating a balanced diet everyday and you have the food available when you need to cook it!

You might think $50 for a piece of premium lamb seems expensive, but when that lamb feeds a family a beautiful roast meal and then leftovers are used for sandwiches, salads and wraps for most of the week, maybe even another dinner, then the bone popped in the stockpot to make a stock for a delicious soup or sauce - that piece of lamb is actually a bargain! And NO it doesn't get boring, that roast lamb could be a couple of chickens, beef or pork. I have not met a child yet who does not enjoy a roast with all the roast veggies.

Knowing I am cooking a roast on the Sunday night is a good opportunity for me to be in the kitchen for a few hours and get a few other bits and pieces ready to take the load off the busy school days. I will have myself organised for a bit of a Sunday afternoon cook up, and when we were commuting 3 plus hours return from Eaglehawk Neck, leaving just before 7 am to Hobart 6 days a week, with activities every night and arriving home after 9pm for 6 years, believe me it helped!

We have a family of five, including three children that eat like teenagers. I usually cook a 2-3 kilo roast on a Sunday. We will eat approximately one third to a half on Sunday and we are left with the remainder for the rest of the week. Stored in a sealed container, the leftovers will keep for 3-4 days.

My favourite is roast lamb, but I also like to mix it up. You could cook:

- 2 chickens
- 3 kilos pork
- 3 kilos beef

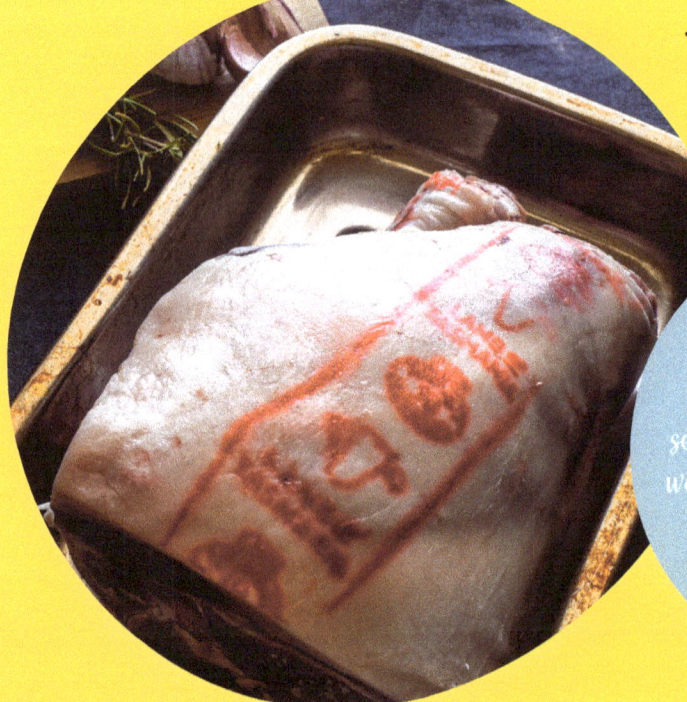

A 3-4 kilo premium leg of lamb for $50 may seem expensive, but when you see how far it goes towards your weekly meals its a bargain. What could you buy for $50 worth of takeaways - not much!

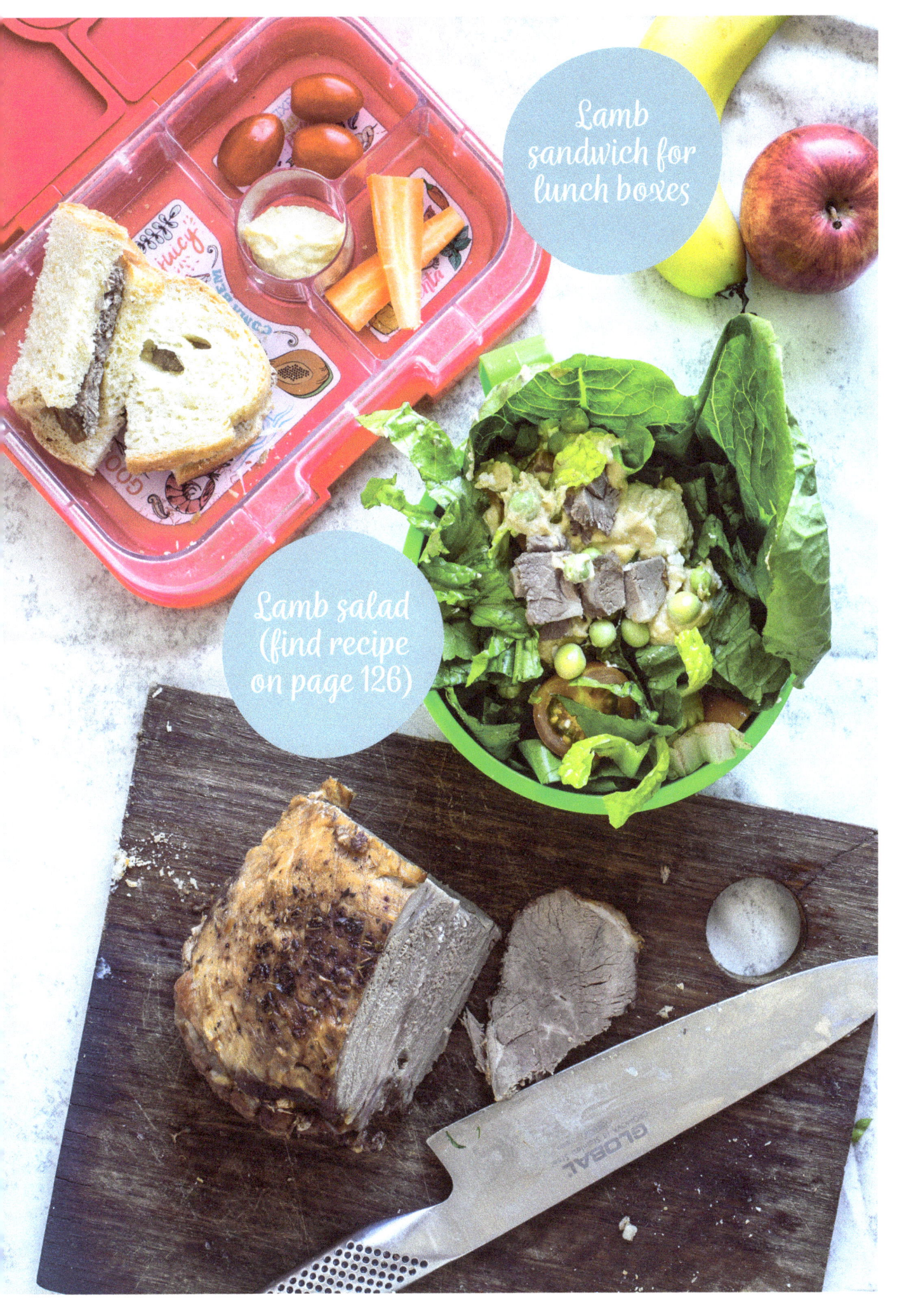

Lamb sandwich for lunch boxes

Lamb salad (find recipe on page 126)

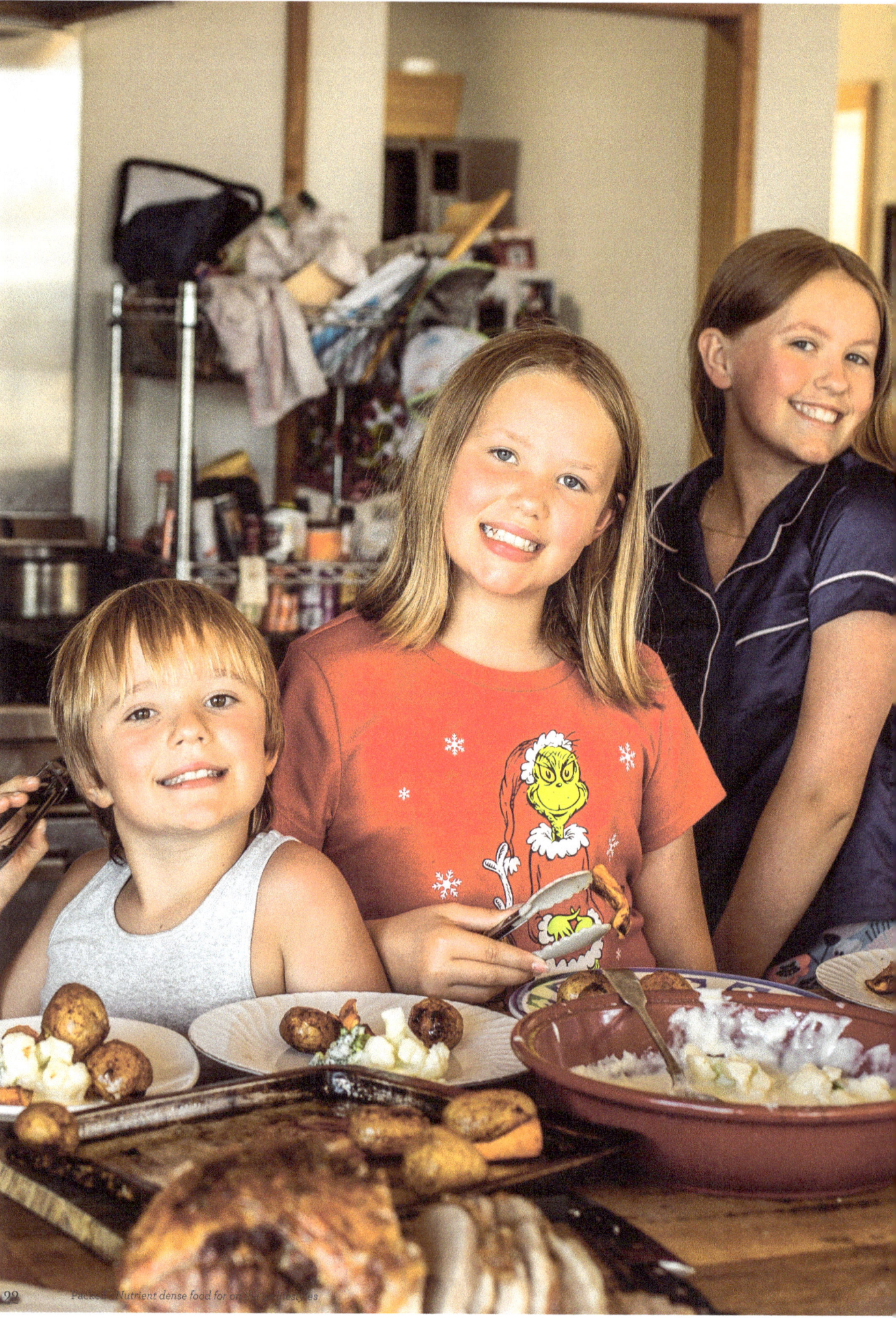

To find ideas on how to season your roast see page 27.

Week one whilst cooking my Sunday roast I might:

- Pop on a soup and freeze down 6 single portions.
- Make a chilli con carne in the thermocooker that is enough for 4 family meals, one in the fridge for Wednesday night to go with nachos and 3 in the freezer.
- Marinate the chicken. I will cook Monday night to roll sushi Tuesday am to pack for Tuesday dinner.
- Cook extra veggies like roast pumpkin and make a tzatziki as this will go with the leftover lamb for a salad for Mondays cold packed dinner.
- Make a slice for a after school snack.
- Make a stack of wraps to go in the freezer.
- Make some scrolls for the freezer for something quick to grab out for a packed lunch.

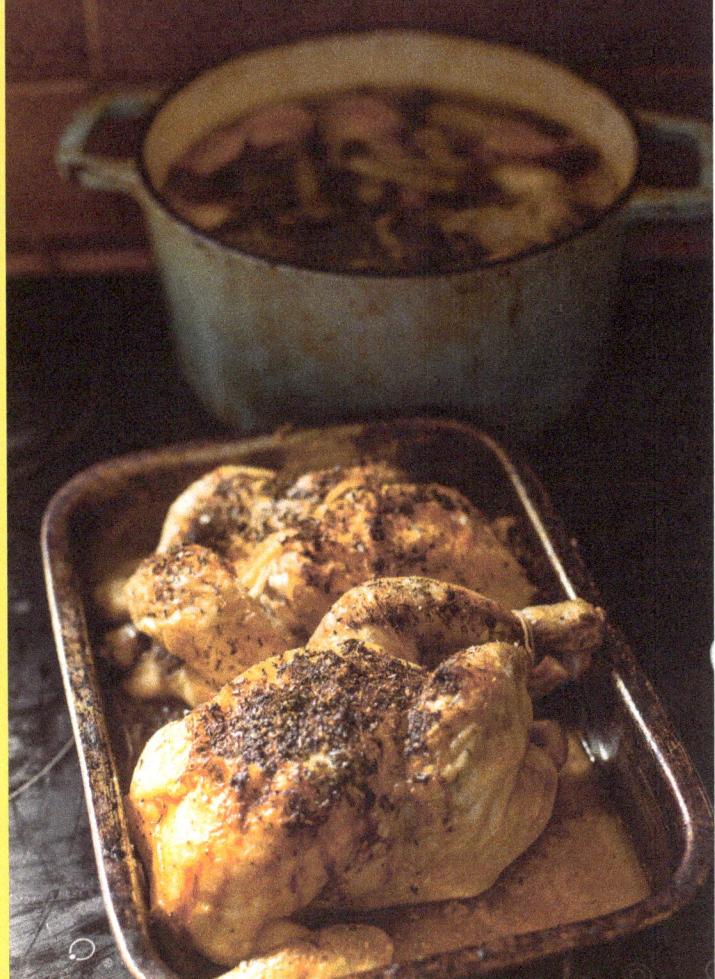

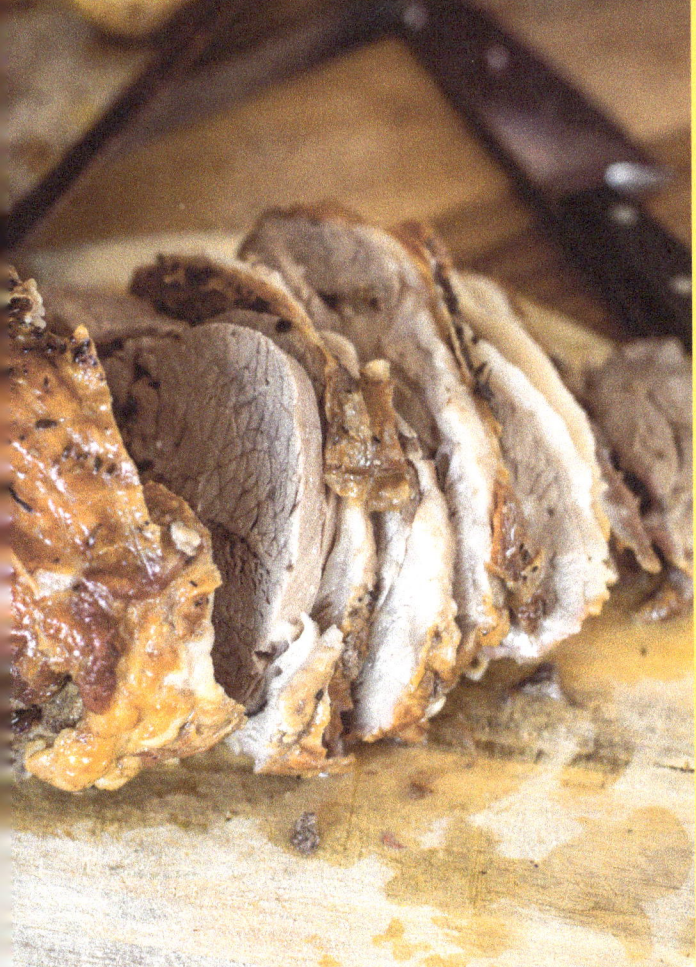

Week two I could be too busy with a weekend retreat. This is when I call on my freezer reserves.

Week three whilst cooking my Sunday roast I might:

- Cook a bolognaise for 4 family meals - one for Wednesday night dinner and 3 for the freezer
- Prepare the pork for sichaun peppered salads on Tuesday
- Marinate the chicken to cook Tuesday night for Wednesdays schnitzel bowls for a cold packed dinner
- Make apricot balls for after school

So I keep ahead and it is just a few things every week!

Doing something to help make the next day or a future day easier always helps! And it really is easy when you are organised!

The Basics

Salad Dressings

Traditionally a salad dressing is one third vinegar or acid like lemon juice to two thirds oil. There are some lovely vinegars available to buy such as pomegranate and shallot, easy to whip up in a dressing just pour into a container with the oil each day. Other ideas are red wine, white wine, apple cider. Always use a certified extra virgin olive oil that will not be faulted and be very flavoursome. Use a mild oil for a dressing like the pomegranate vinegar and something robust for your spicy dressings. Some robust extra virgin olive oils are great as a dressing on there own they have plenty of flavour. Infused and agrumato oils add extra flavours as well and there are interesting flavours to buy. I love a lemon agrumato oil on leafy greens with fish, simple and delicious.

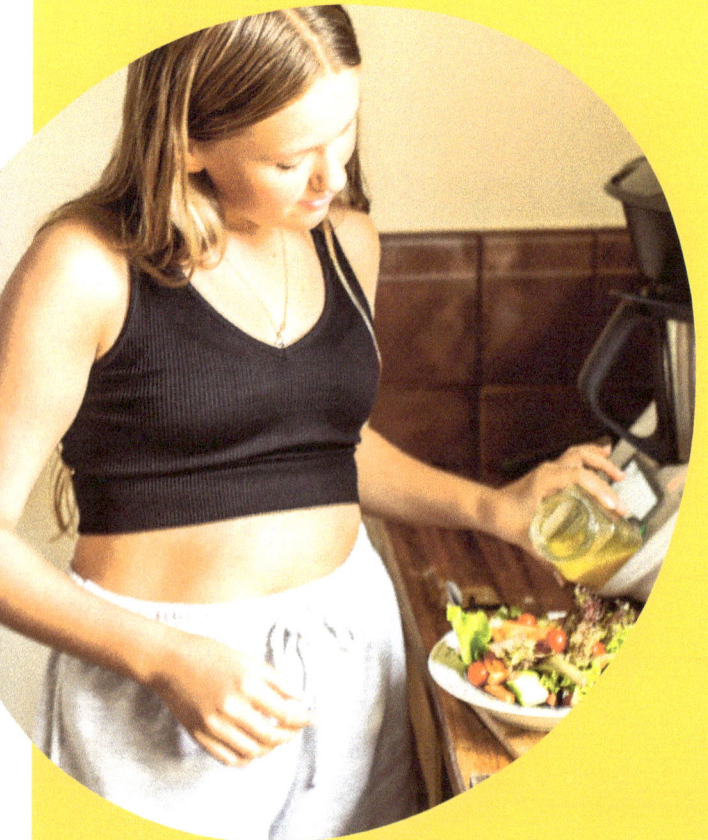

SOY BALSAMIC

1 tablespoon soy sauce

1 tablespoon balsamic

2 tablespoons extra virgin olive oil

HONEY MUSTARD

1 teaspoon Dijon mustard

1 teaspoon honey

1 tablespoon white wine vinegar

2 tablespoons extra virgin olive oil

LEMON AND OREGANO

1 tablespoon lemon juice

2 tablespoon extra virgin olive oil

1 tablespoon oregano

1 clove crushed garlic

ROSEMARY AND GARLIC

1 tablespoon red wine vinegar

2 tablespoons extra virgin olive oil

1 tablespoon rosemary

1 clove garlic crushed

Mayonnaise/Aioli

1 egg

½ tsp dijon mustard

1 tablespoon white vinegar

pinch salt

pinch pepper

200ml (approx.) extra virgin olive oil

Traditionally we just use the yolk to use mayo but then what do we do with the whites? For home cooking I just use the whole egg and it works out fine!

Either use your thermocooker, food processor or a bowl, whisk and fast moving arm. Mix the eggs, mustard and vinegar together and whilst whisking fast, pour the oil in a slow drizzle until all combined and thick. Season with the salt and pepper.

TARTARE

Replace the vinegar with 1 tablespoon lemon juice and when the mayonnaise is made add one tablespoon of chopped gherkins and 1 tablespoon chopped capers

GARLIC AIOLI

Add 2 crushed cloves of garlic to the eggs and vinegar before starting, or whole garlic cloves in the thermocooker at the start with the eggs.

CAPER BALSAMIC

Substitute the white vinegar with balsamic vinegar and add 2 tablespoons of chopped capers.

DILL MAYONNAISE

Add 2 tablespoons of dill to the mayonnaise.

SEAFOOD SAUCE

Add 1 tablespoon tomato sauce, ¼ teaspoon Worcestershire sauce and a few drops to your liking of tobasco sauce to the mayonnaise.

HONEY MUSTARD MAYONNAISE

This one is awesome with salmon or chicken! Add 2 tablespoons honey and an extra teaspoon of dijon to the eggs and vinegar before adding the oil.

Garlic Pizza

This recipe makes 2 large garlic pizzas. Use this simple base for 2 large pizzas of your liking. I love baking bread and I love making my own pizzas for the family. My kids can choose the toppings and I know exactly what we are eating. There are so many different ideas for pizza toppings. Garlic, ham and pineapple and BBQ chicken are always popular in our house. Avoid the jars of tomato sauce for your pizza base as they are full of sugar and not tasty. It is much better to make your own with fresh or tinned tomatoes, onion, garlic, basil and oregano.

500 grams flour

1 teaspoon yeast

1 teaspoon salt

1 teaspoon sugar

300ml - 320ml water

robust extra virgin olive oil

sea salt

2 tablespoons garlic

mozzarella or tasty cheese

sea salt

Heat the oven to 200°C.

To make the dough knead all ingredients well, I use the thermocooker or you can use any mixer or knead by hand on the bench for around 10 minutes to produce a smooth firm dough.

Cover and leave to rise in a warm position until the dough has doubled in size. Knock the dough back down and divide into 2 and roll into tight balls.

Roll the dough out into large (around 30cm diameter) pizza bases and lay the bases on a baking tray rubbed with some of the extra virgin olive oil, and then sprinkle on the crushed garlic and cheese drizzle with the oil and a sprinkle of sea salt.

If you like a thin base be ready to cook your pizza straightaway. If you like it thicker leave it to rise after you have put your toppings on.

Bake for around 15-20 minutes or until golden brown and cooked through.

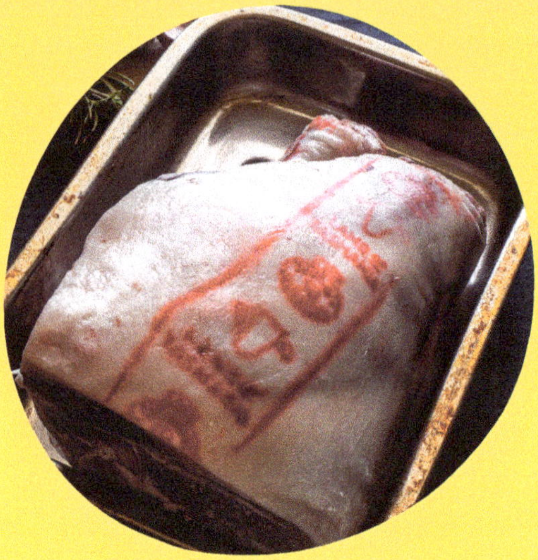

Roast Lamb

Lamb leg

4 sprigs rosemary

3 cloves garlic

REAL GRAVY

2 tablespoons plain flour

3 cups beef stock

1 tablespoon chutney or plum sauce etc

Salt and pepper

6 cups vegetables to roast such as pumpkin, parsnip, carrot, beetroot, onion, sweet potato and potato

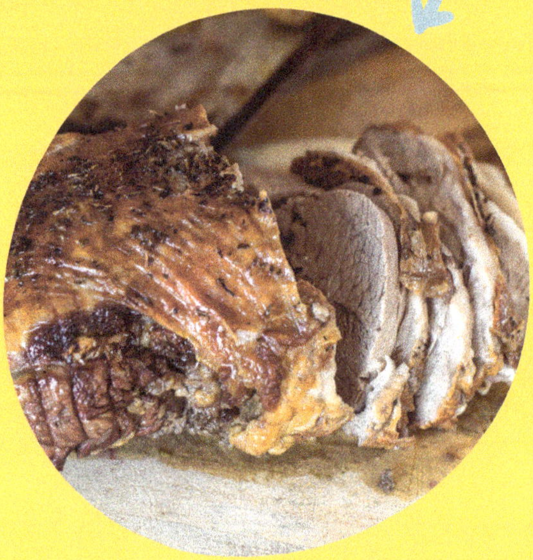

Heat the oven to 180°C.

Make small cuts in the lamb preferably under skin, between sinew so not to cut the actual flesh and insert rosemary, garlic and lemon. Put the lamb in a baking dish and cook for 1 hour. Peel and cut vegetables into 3 cm chunks .

Take the lamb out and put in on a rack, put the vegetable in the baking tray and the lamb back on top and bake for a further 30 minutes. Now the lamb should be ready (for medium rare to medium) to come out and wrapped in foil to rest while the vegetables finish cooking for about 10 minutes.

To make the gravy take the veggies out of the tray, put the tray on the hot plate on low heat and put the flour in, cook this to it is brown then add stock and chutney and season with salt and pepper and cook for about 10 minutes continuing stirring.

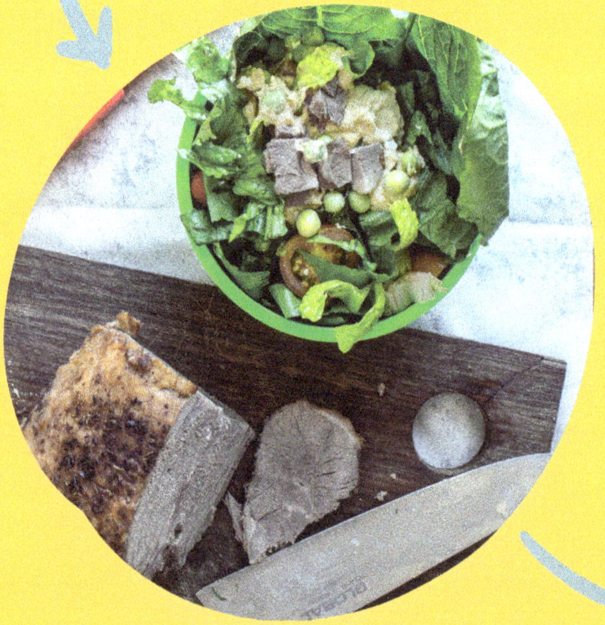

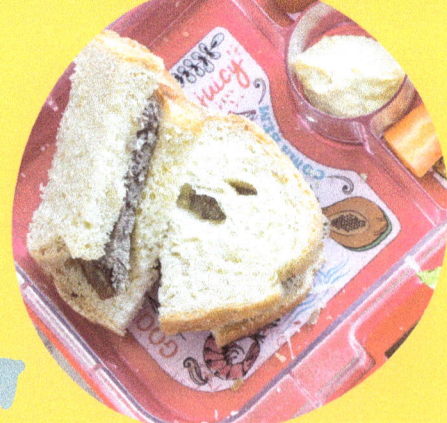

Lemon, Garlic and Herb Roasted Chicken

1 lemon juice and zest

2 tablespoons tarragon

1 tablespoon sage

1 tablespoon rosemary

1 tablespoon parsley

1 tablespoon thyme

2 cloves garlic

olive oil

1 chicken

salt and pepper

vegetables to roast a selection of pumpkin, potato, sweet potato, carrot, parsnip or beetroot.

Heat the oven to 180°C.

Chop the herbs, crush the garlic and mix together with the lemon, oil and salt and pepper. Rub the herb mix into the chicken and put on a rack above the peeled vegetables that are in a baking dish cut into approximately 3cm pieces and rubbed with oil. Bake for about 1 hour (for a small chicken) or until cooked through and the vegetables are cooked too.

SEASONING IDEAS

CHICKEN

Drizzle robust extra virgin olive over and sprinkle one teaspoon of each smoked paprika, oregano, tarragon, white pepper and sea salt This is our standard seasoning for chickens for meat for sandwiches, wraps and salads with the bones cooked up into a delicious broth.

BEEF

For a simple beef seasoning rub the piece of beef with a few tablespoons of seeded mustard or make a mix of preserved lemon, horseradish and fresh herbs.

LAMB

Garlic and rosemary popped into slits in the lamb and drizzled with extra virgin olive oil or mix together a few tablespoons of honey and mustard to rub over the meat.

PORK

Tips to get the best crackle.

Use fresh pork! Rub a few spoonfuls of salt into the skin a few hours before cooking, this will remove some moisture. Wipe dry and then rub fresh salt into the skin with a drizzle of oil. Start the roast in the oven as hot as you can get the oven.

Stock/Bone Broth

A good stock is the essential for a lot of meals. Sauce and gravy need a meat stock, laksa, soups, risotto, casseroles all benefit from a vegetable, meat, chicken or fish stock. Stocks are extremely easy and economical to make, and if you use the slow cooker they are don't need any attention. I also only use off-cuts for stocks and you can collect these while you are cooking, and keep them in a freezer bag in the freezer ready for when you need to make a stock. These may be the greens and ends from leeks, ends and peels from carrots, end and some peel from onions, ends and some peel from garlic, ends of tomatoes or discarded seeds, stalks from parsley, bacon rind, celery leaves and ends. Sometimes I might need to balance out the off-cuts with some fresh vegetables from the above list. Throw the bones at the end of a roast in the stock too.

If you buy your meat in bulk, for example a side of beef direct from the farm like I like to, you will have bones to use up, or if you fillet whole fish, or ask your fishmonger for some frames, or bone out your own chickens or ask the butcher for some frames and bones.

BEEF STOCK

1 kilo beef bones

500 grams of offcuts such as onions, celery, carrots, leeks, garlic, tomatoes, parley stalks, bacon rinds.

2 bay leaves

5 peppercorns

4 sprigs thyme

1 teaspoon salt

Put all ingredients in a baking tray and bake in a hot oven until browned, about 40 minutes. Put in a large slower cooker and cover with water and simmer on low for 8 hours. Strain, cool in the fridge, remove any fat that has set on top and use or freeze.

CHICKEN STOCK

1 kilo chicken bones - or a whole chicken or drumsticks. If using the whole chicken or drumsticks make sure you keep the meat for the soup

500 grams of offcuts such as onions, celery, carrots, leeks, garlic, tomatoes, parley stalks, bacon rinds.

2 bay leaves

5 peppercorns

4 sprigs thyme

1 teaspoon salt

Put all ingredients in the slow cooker and cover with 4 litres of water and simmer on low for 4 hours. Strain and cool in the fridge, remove any fat that has settled on top and freeze or use.

FISH STOCK

1 kilo fish frames

500 grams of offcuts such as onions, celery, carrots, leeks, garlic, tomatoes, parley stalks, bacon rinds.

2 bay leaves

5 peppercorns

4 sprigs of thyme

1 teaspoon salt

Put all ingredients in a large slow cooker and cover with 4 litres of water and cook for 1 hour on the low setting. Leave to cool before straining to let the flavours infuse.

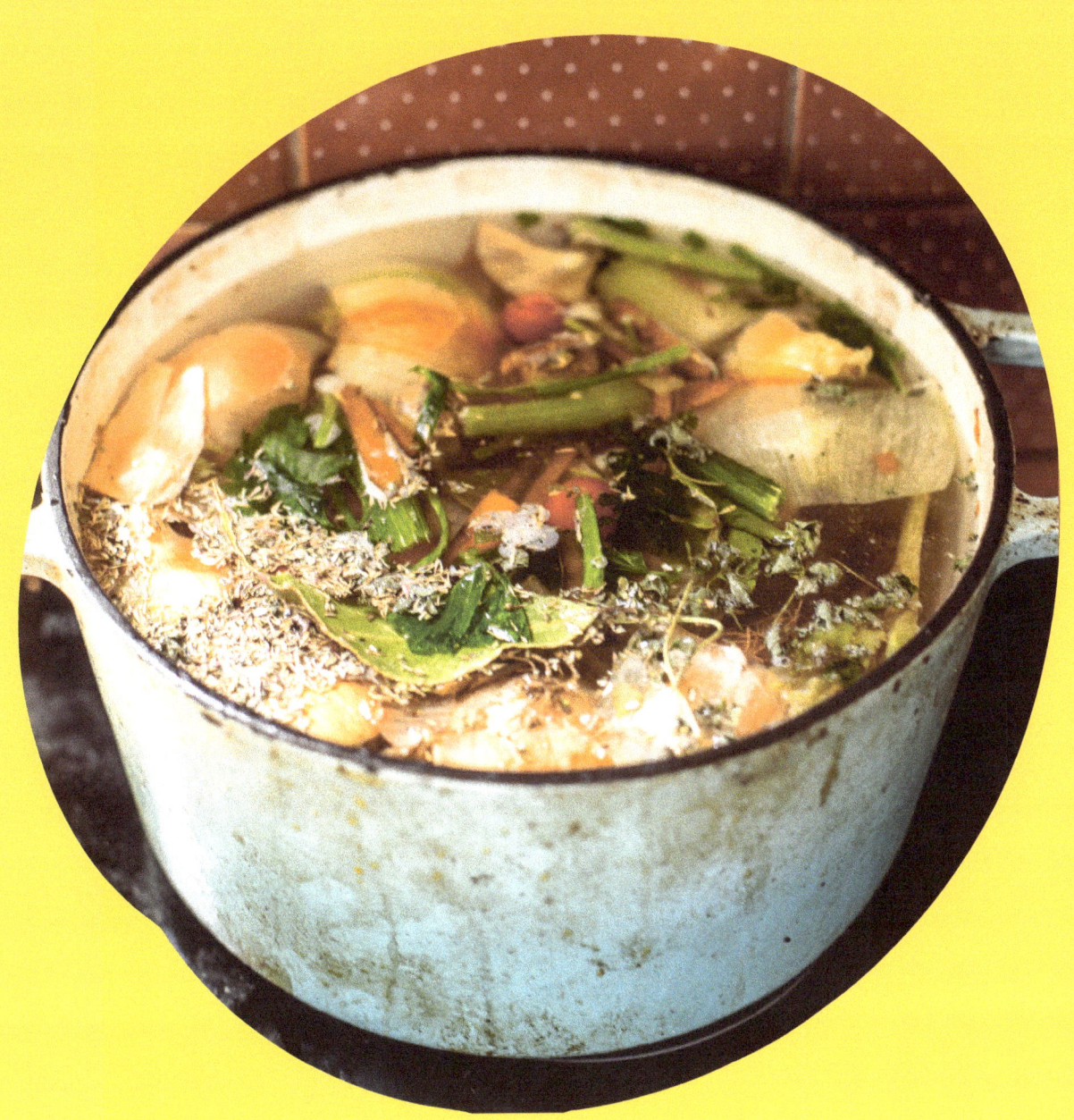

TO TURN YOUR STOCK INTO A SAUCE

To make what is now commonly called jus, but I was taught it's called demi-glaze, from a beef or chicken stock take two litres of stock and add 100 grams of tomato paste and 300ml red wine and reduce its volume by half by placing it in a heavy base pot and leaving it on a low simmer. Season with salt and pepper.

Ideas of flavours that you can add to your jus are sage or other herbs, quince paste, port, onion jam, peppercorns, pepper berries or figs. Or add mushrooms or green peppercorns and a dash of cream for a delicious sauce for your steak.

BROWN RICE COOKED IN STOCK

I cook my brown rice in stock to add in extra nutrients and flavour. It can be stored in the fridge for about 5 days or cooked in bulk and frozen if you have the space. Sometimes when I've made a stock in the slow cooker and its strained I pop the stock and rice back into the slow cooker and cook it in there.

Add one cup brown rice to 3 cups stock and simmer gently covered until the rice is cooked. Eat cold in salads or on the side of curry and other wet dishes.

Chicken Ceaser

SERVES 4

This is not overly time consuming but it does require a little bit of effort. You can do this the day before and it is a delicious meal that would be worthy of a great café (this dressing has been on many restaurant menus I have worked in). This is a very good example of a fairly healthy filling, high protein and good fat dinner that just can get destroyed commercially with cheap and nasty ingredients that can be so bad for you! Think of the effort as saving yourself at least $25!

I also serve this with Tassal Salmon, smoked quail or chunks of roasted meat.

600 grams chicken thighs

4 slices bread

1 tablespoon vinegar

60 grams parmesan

2 rashers bacon

2 baby cos

4 eggs

extra virgin olive oil and teaspoon butter to cook croutons

DRESSING

1 egg

1 small clove garlic

leaves of fresh or dried basil

cracked pepper

2 anchovies

extra virgin olive oil (approx. 70 ml)

Heat the oven to 180°C.

To cook the chicken and bacon: Coat the thighs in a drizzle of oil and place in a baking tray. Remove the rind from the bacon and slice into about 3mm batons and place in the same tray as the chicken. Bake for around 20 minutes or until cooked chicken is cooked through. If your bacon is not as crispy as you prefer take the chicken out of the pan and continue cooking your bacon until it is crispy. Cool bacon on paper.

Boil the eggs for 7 minutes for a not-too-soft boiled egg. Cool and peel.

To make the dressing: In a thermocooker, food processor or a bowl (and whisk with a fast-moving arm), add the egg and vinegar, basil, anchovies, cracked pepper and peeled garlic clove (crushed if using your arm) and while blending on a high speed drizzle the oil in a very slow-moving stream until you have a thick dressing.

To make the croutons: Dice the bread in 1-2cm cubes. Heat an oven proof pan over low heat, I like to use a mix of butter and oil, both for flavour and butter for crunchiness and oil to stop it burning. Heat the oil to a medium heat in a heavy based pan and then sauté the bread in one layer, once all the croutons are coated in fat put the pan in the oven for around 8 minutes until the croutons are crisp. Cool on kitchen paper.

Wash and spin the lettuce, shave the parmesan and assemble and dress the salad as close to serving time as possible.

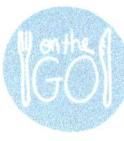

This is one of our favourite cold packed dinners. I have the chicken, bacon, croutons and dressing made, lettuce washed and parmesan shaved the evening before. (Leave croutons out on the bench overnight - do no refrigerate or they will be soggy). In 4 containers in the morning I put in the lettuce and in a pile to the side the chicken, bacon, egg, parmesan and then keep the dressing and croutons to throw in when we are about to eat.

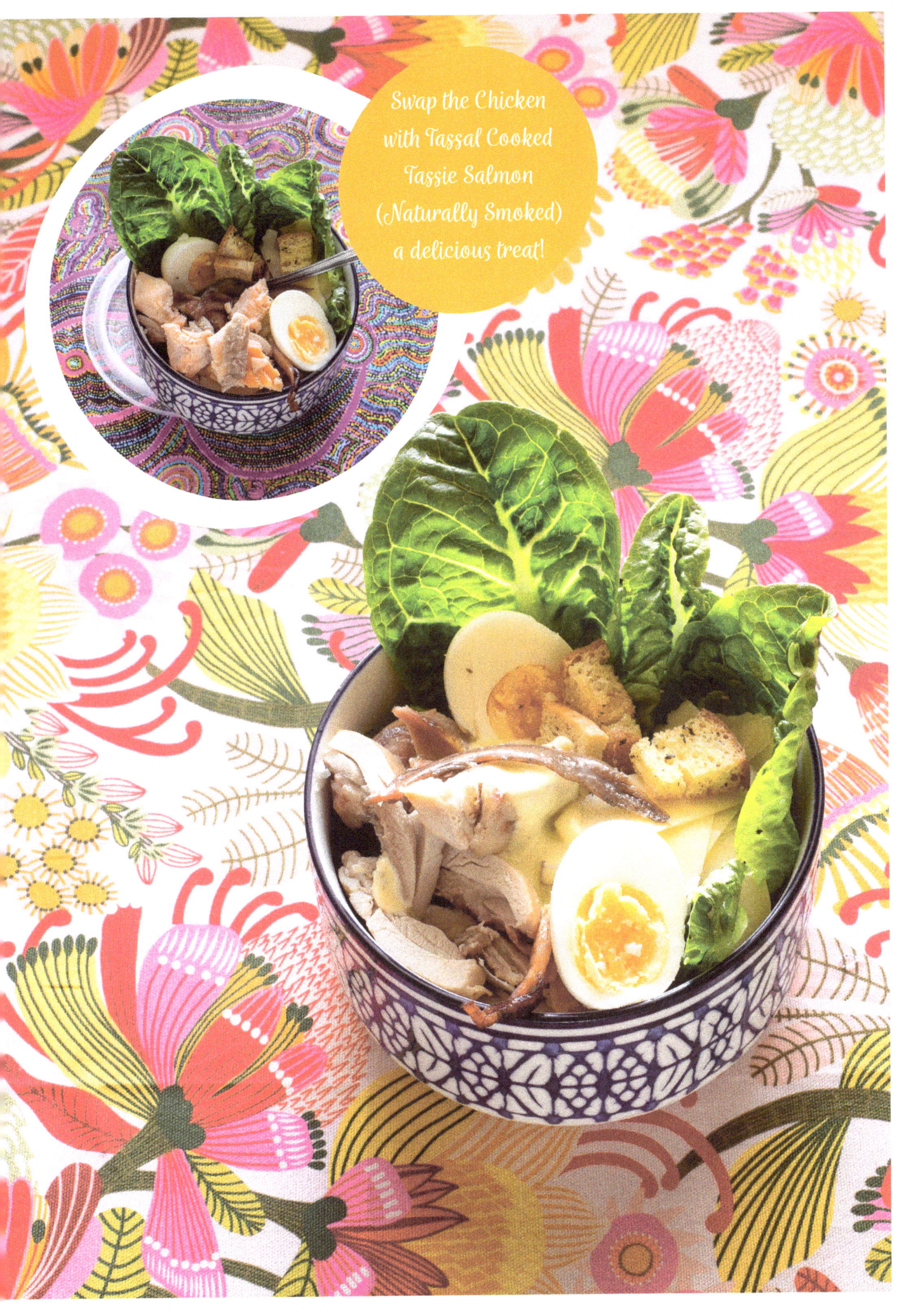

Swap the Chicken with Tassal Cooked Tassie Salmon (Naturally Smoked) a delicious treat!

Cauliflower and Broccoli Mac and Cheese

SERVES 4-6

Served in a food container that keeps food hot, with some leftover chunks of roasted meat or a tin of fish, this ticks a few food groups at lunch. Or its great as a quick one tray dinner on the side of a baked piece of fish, chicken, chop or steak. Or you could add in salmon or chicken thigh when baking. Choose a good quality pasta or use your favourite GF (Gluten Free) pasta and substitute brown rice flour for a GF version.

2 cups macaroni (cooked to packet instructions)

2 cups cauliflower florets

2 cups broccoli florets

CHEESE SAUCE

600ml milk

30 grams butter

20ml extra virgin olive oil

60 grams flour

½ teaspoon Dijon mustard

100 grams cheddar cheese

40 grams parmesan

salt

pepper

parsley fresh or dried

Heat the oven to 180°C.

To make the sauce, I make it easily in my thermocooker, but you can use a pot and spoon and a fast-moving arm. Melt the butter and oil, add the flour and stir for a few minutes while the flour cooks. Then pour the milk in slowly and cook for around five minutes until thick and cooked through. Add mustard and season with salt and pepper. Add grated cheeses and parsley and mix well.

Cook the pasta to the packet directions and steam the cauliflower and broccoli florets until cooked through. Mix the pasta with the broccoli and cauliflower and lay in a baking tray and cover with the sauce. Bake for 15 minutes until golden brown on top.

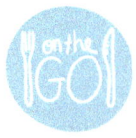

For on the go, have the tray prepped and ready to pop in the oven at breakfast to heat through and transfer to warmed thermos. Or I pre-cook and simply scoop and microwave for the thermos.

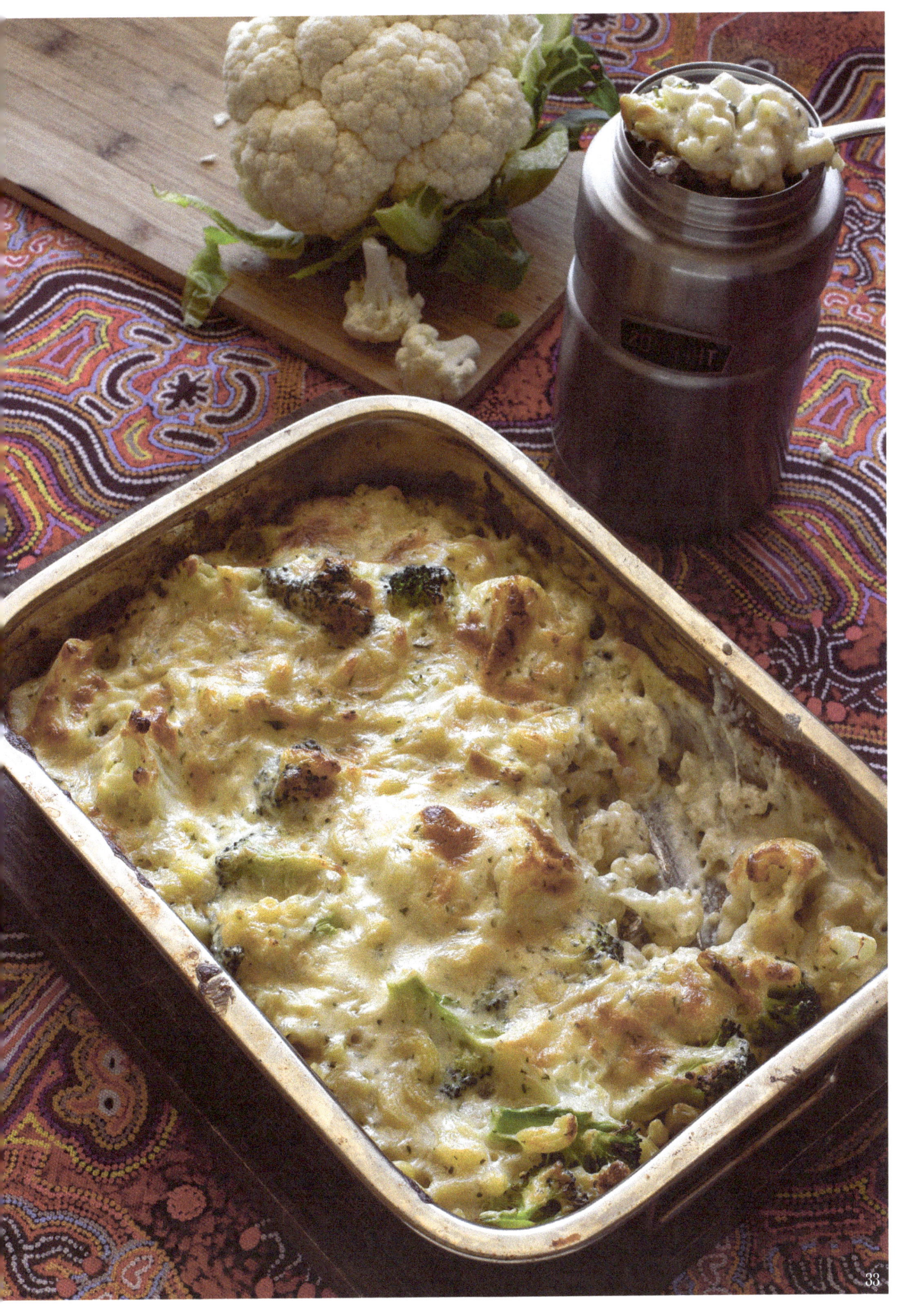

Asian Flavoured Schnitzel Bowl

SERVES 4

Although the ingredient list here is looking long this is an easy meal to whip up when you are in the habit of having homemade mayo in the fridge or have figured out how to quickly whip it up. And you have your own dressings made or the products easily on hand. Sometimes I simply chuck the crumbs into the marinated chicken to cook the chicken and this works fine but I have added the proper crumbing steps into the recipes for a really great crispy chicken. The thighs can be frozen once cooked to make this even easier.

4 chicken thighs

1 tablespoon soy sauce

1 tablespoon honey

1 egg

1 cup flour

1 cup breadcrumbs

extra virgin olive oil

2 sticks celery

2 cups cabbage

1 cup bean sprouts

2 carrots

4 spring onions

2 cups lettuce

1 cup brown rice cooked in stock and cooled

SALAD DRESSING

½ teaspoon honey

1 teaspoon soy

1 teaspoon balsamic

2 tablespoons extra virgin olive oil

MAYONNAISE

1 egg

1 tablespoon vinegar

½ teaspoon Dijon mustard

½ teaspoon honey

extra virgin olive oil (approx. 70 ml)

EXTRAS TO SERVE

kecap manis (thick soy)
and chopped chillies

Mix the honey and soy together and leave the thighs to marinate, overnight ideally but for a hour or so at least.

Heat the oven to 170°C.

Crumb the chicken by cracking the egg into a bowl and whisking it up with a fork and then dipping each thigh into the flour, shaking off excess flour, then dipping the thigh in egg and then dipping each thigh in the bread crumbs.

To make the mayo, use a blender or food processor to combine the whole egg, Dijon mustard, honey, vinegar and a sprinkle of salt and pepper. With the motor running, slowly add the oil in a steady drizzle to create a thick, creamy emulsion.

Mix the dressing ingredients together in a jar.

Wash, spin and shred the lettuce. Add the shredded cabbage, julienned carrot, sliced spring onion, sprouts, rice and celery and dress just before serving.

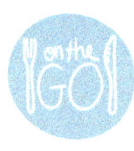

To serve on the go, I pack the salad not dressed, with the chicken sliced up on top. I put the dressings in separate container, to dress when eating. This can be packed before 6am in a cooler bag on ice for the day, for a delicious 6pm dinner.

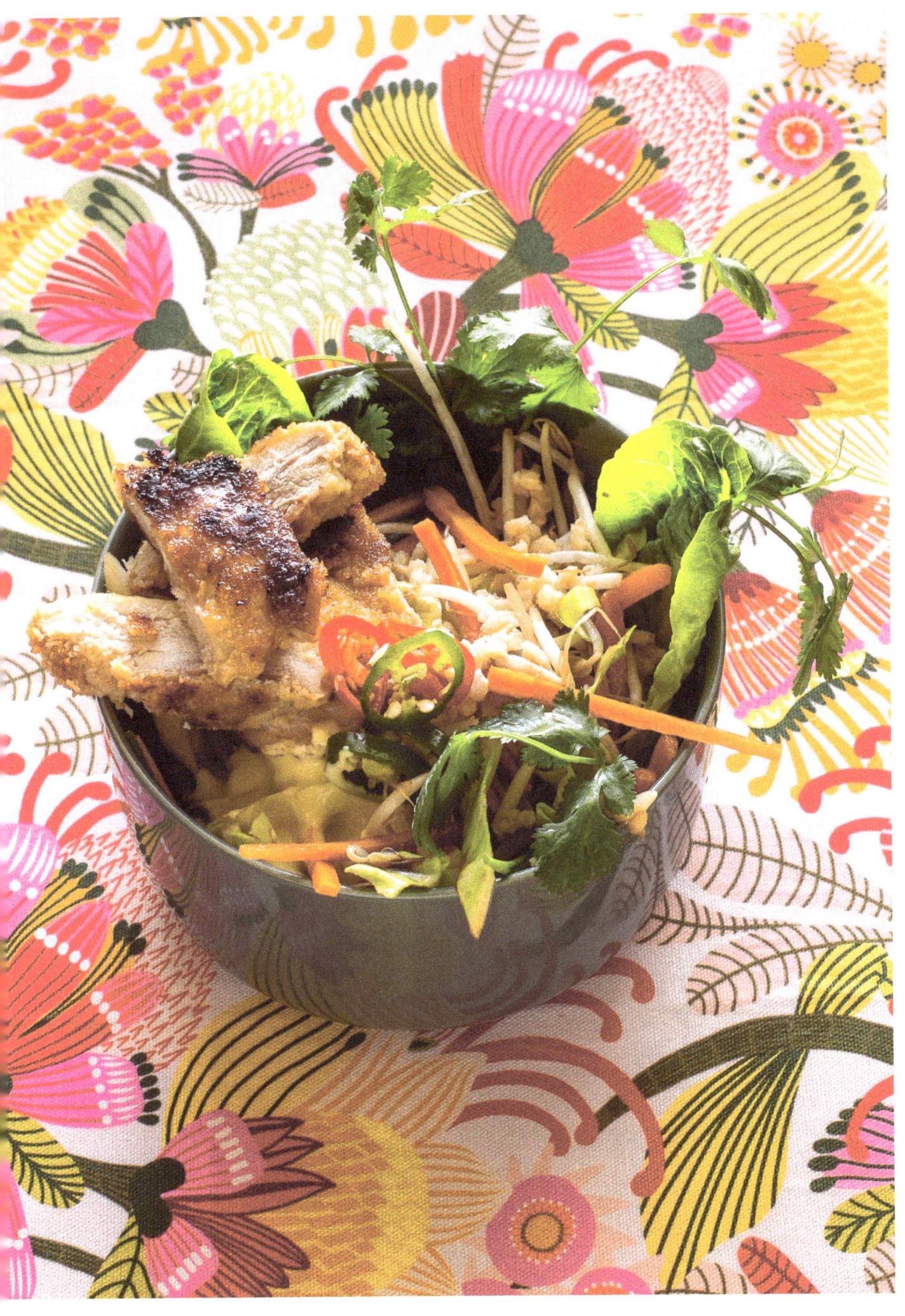

Apple and Carrot Breakie Muffins

MAKES 18 MUFFINS OF ABOUT 2 LARGE TABLESPOON SCOOPS OF BATTER

These are handy grab and go breakfast option when I have let the kids sleep in as late as possible after a later night of after school activities or events. They freeze well so can simply be taken out of the freezer the night before or warmed quickly in the oven. Serve with lashings of butter or cream cheese beaten with a little honey.

2 medium carrots

2 apples

1 teaspoon cinnamon

2 tablespoons honey

3 eggs

1 cup oats

2 cups self raising flour

½ cup raisins

½ cup dates

½ cup extra virgin olive oil

1 cup almonds

Heat the oven to 180°C.

Grate the apples and carrots (or chop them in the thermocooker).

Mix all ingredients well together.

Pour into muffin trays and bake for 20 minutes.

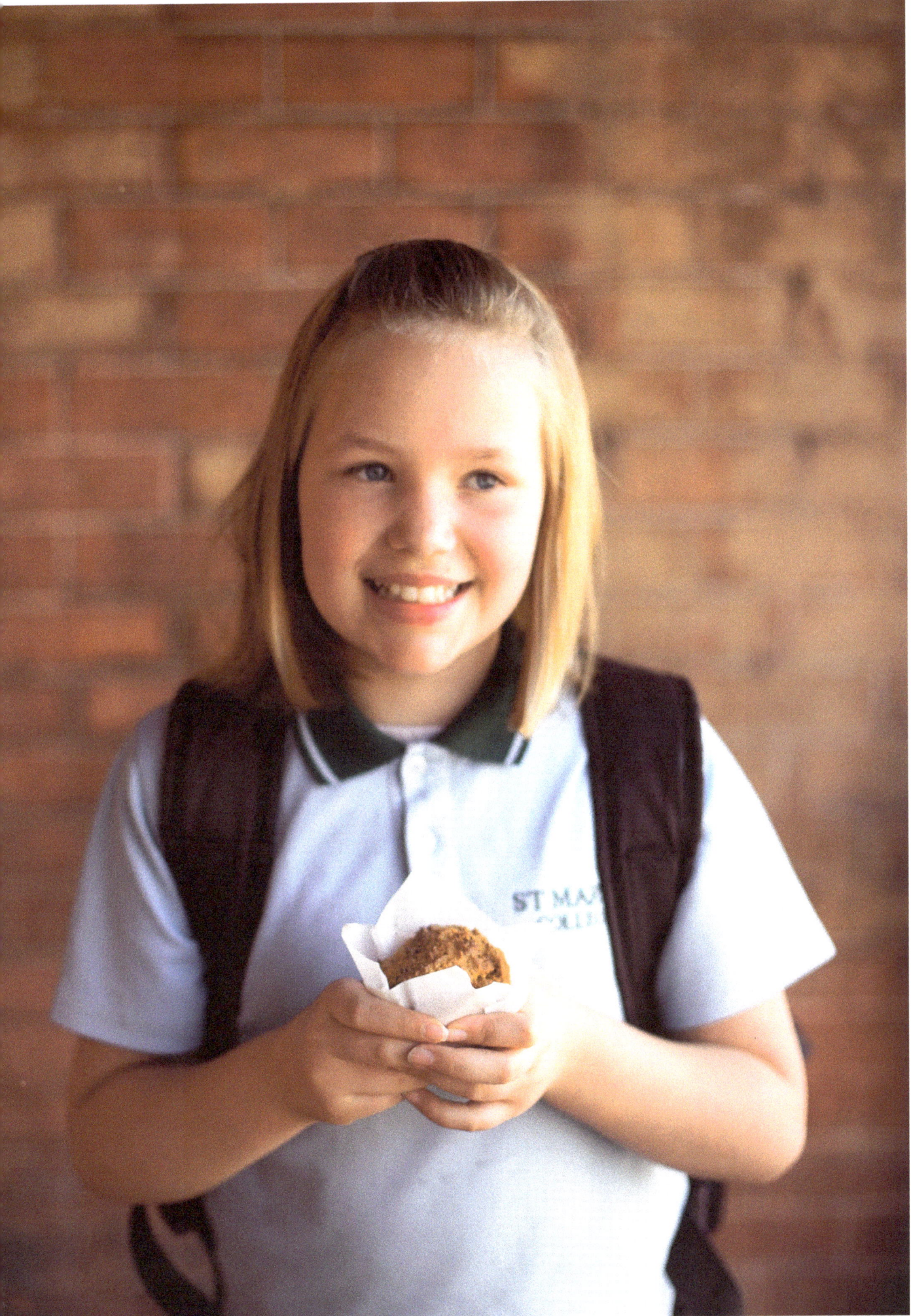

Tropic Co Prawn, Broccoli and Apple Salad with a Honey and Mustard Dressing

SERVES 4

This is a simple and convenient way to whip up a salad. Serve this salad with steamed or roasted chicken, a few boiled eggs, chunks of leftover roasted meats, smoked or cold steamed salmon or fish, or on the side of a steak or lamb chop. Serve with some nuts or cheese, walnuts and blue cheese work superbly, or on its own. Prawns may seem like a luxury but when we look at our comparison to takeaway, they are quite affordable. Frozen prawns from the Salmon Shop Salamanca and other main grocery stores and fishmongers make an affordable super quick to whip up delicious healthy packed dinner, this simple salad take 5 minutes max!!

800 grams whole cooked Tropic Co prawns

1 large head of broccoli

2 sticks celery

2 apples

2 carrots

1 cup cabbage

handful parsley

2 tablespoons robust extra virgin olive oil

2 tablespoons dijon mustard

2 tablespoons honey

sea salt

cracked pepper

To make the salad simply cut the veggies into chunks, pop all the ingredients in the thermocooker or blender and chop slowly for a few seconds for a chunky salad. Alternatively grate or finely chop each vegetable and mix well together. Peel prawns by removing the shells and place them on top.

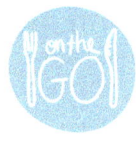

With the robust veggies in this salad it lasts well for at least 12 hours, or even the day before packed in a cooler bag with ice.

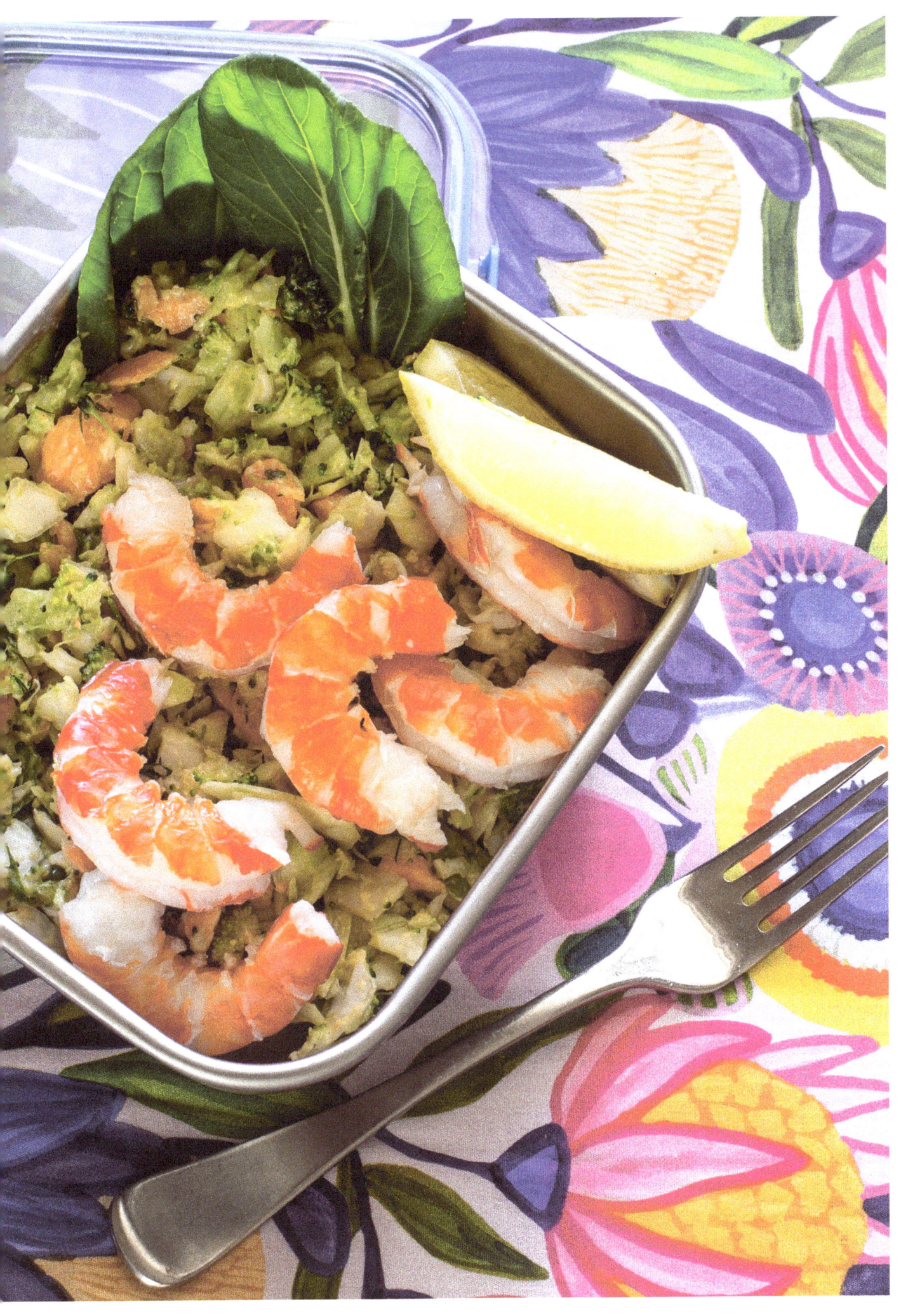

Potato and Bacon Salad

SERVES 4

Serve with a piece of cooled baked salmon or chicken, roast meat, tins of fish or smoked meats or simply on its own.

4 large pinkeye potatoes
(or another waxy potato variety)

2 rashers bacon

4 eggs

20 chives

2 tablespoons mayonnaise (see basics)

2 tablespoons sour cream

4 cups spinach leaves

2 cups peas

½ teaspoon cracked pepper

Scrub the potatoes well and dice into 2cm pieces and place in a small pot, cover with cold water and bring to a gentle boil for around 20 minutes or until cooked through. In the same pot (pop them in after the potatoes have been cooking for about 12 minutes) or another pot, boil eggs for 7 minutes for a not too soft boiled egg.

Trim the rind from the bacon, slice into 4mm pieces and pan fry over a medium heat until crispy.

Mix the cooled potatoes, egg and bacon with the mayo, sour cream, chopped chives, pepper, peas and spinach.

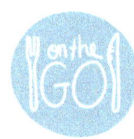

Have your potatoes, eggs and bacon cooked and cooled the day before so on a busy morning you just need to mix it together. BUT do not mix the spinach leaves through as they will wilt if dressed. So, mix everything else well and put the spinach in another container or in a pile on the top of the salad in the same container to mix through just before eating. If you are using frozen peas keep them frozen to help keep the salad cold for the day. Pack in a cooler bag with ice for the day.

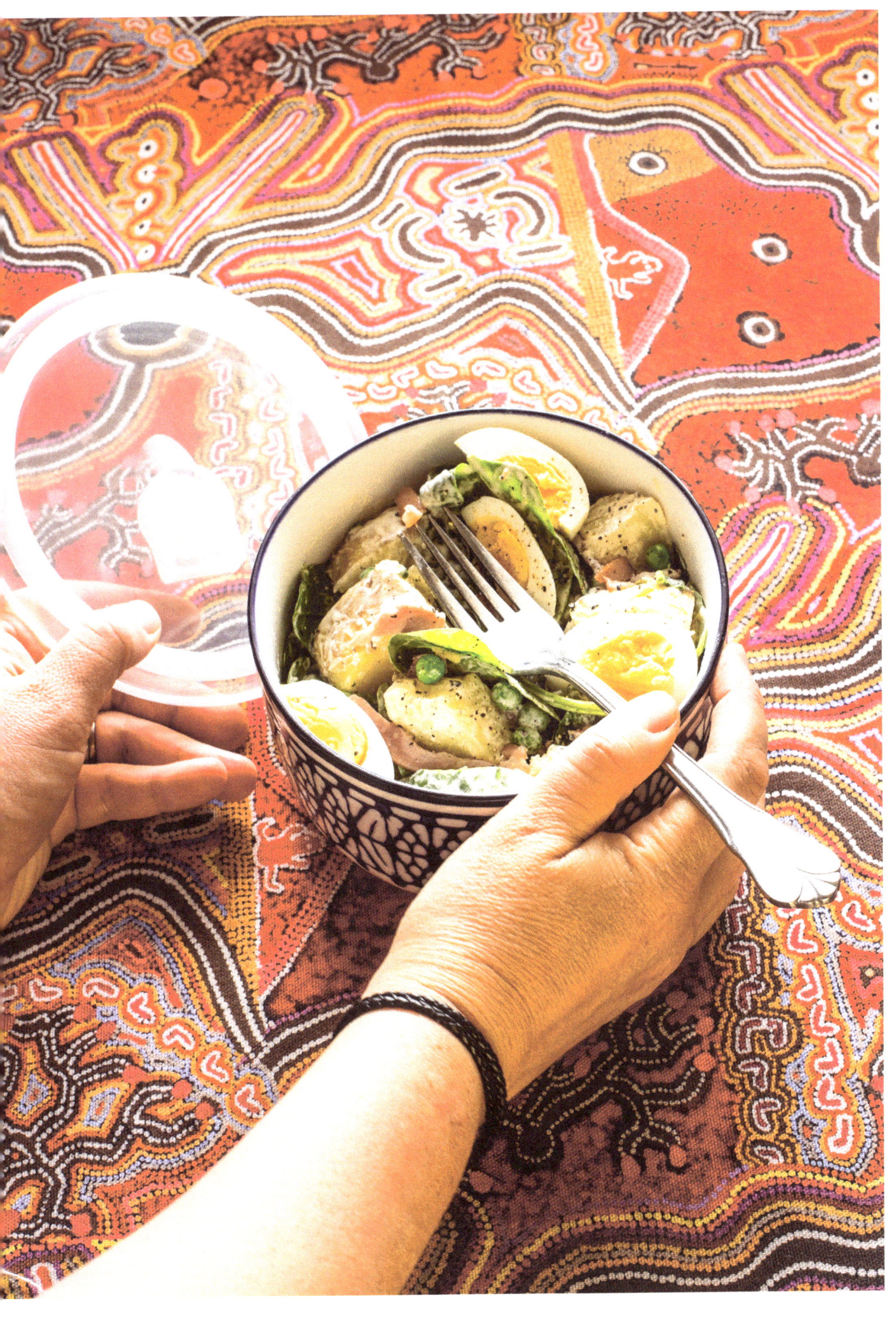

Mexican Pulled Beef

MAKES ENOUGH FOR 2 FAMILY MEALS

On the rare occasion we do buy a takeaway meal and my fussiest says "I love this meat I could eat it every day", I will put A LOT of effort into making a recipe that she loves. This beef is super handy and freezes well to defrost. Add beans and corn to serve with nachos, tacos, wraps, enchilada bakes and more.

1 kilo piece beef chuck roast or any stewing steak

1 onion diced

4 garlic cloves minced

1 tablespoon lime juice

1 tablespoon honey

1 teaspoon cinnamon

1 teaspoon turmeric

2 teaspoons cumin

1 teaspoon paprika

2 teaspoons dried oregano

1 teaspoon sea salt plus more to taste

1 teaspoon black pepper

½ teaspoon red chilli flakes

1 tablespoon extra virgin olive oil

I use my slow cooker but you can use a braising dish and a lid with the oven on low at 150°C.

Seal the beef on all sides in a hot pan. Mix all the ingredients together and rub over the beef and place in the slow cooker with 2 cups beef stock. Cook on low for about 5 hours or until you can pull the meat apart with a fork.

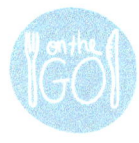

Serve beef with tacos, in nachos or burritos. Pop corn chips in one container and cheese and sauces in others, and the beef in a thermos. Top the warm beef on top of the corn chips to enjoy a delicious satisfying lunch or dinner on the go!

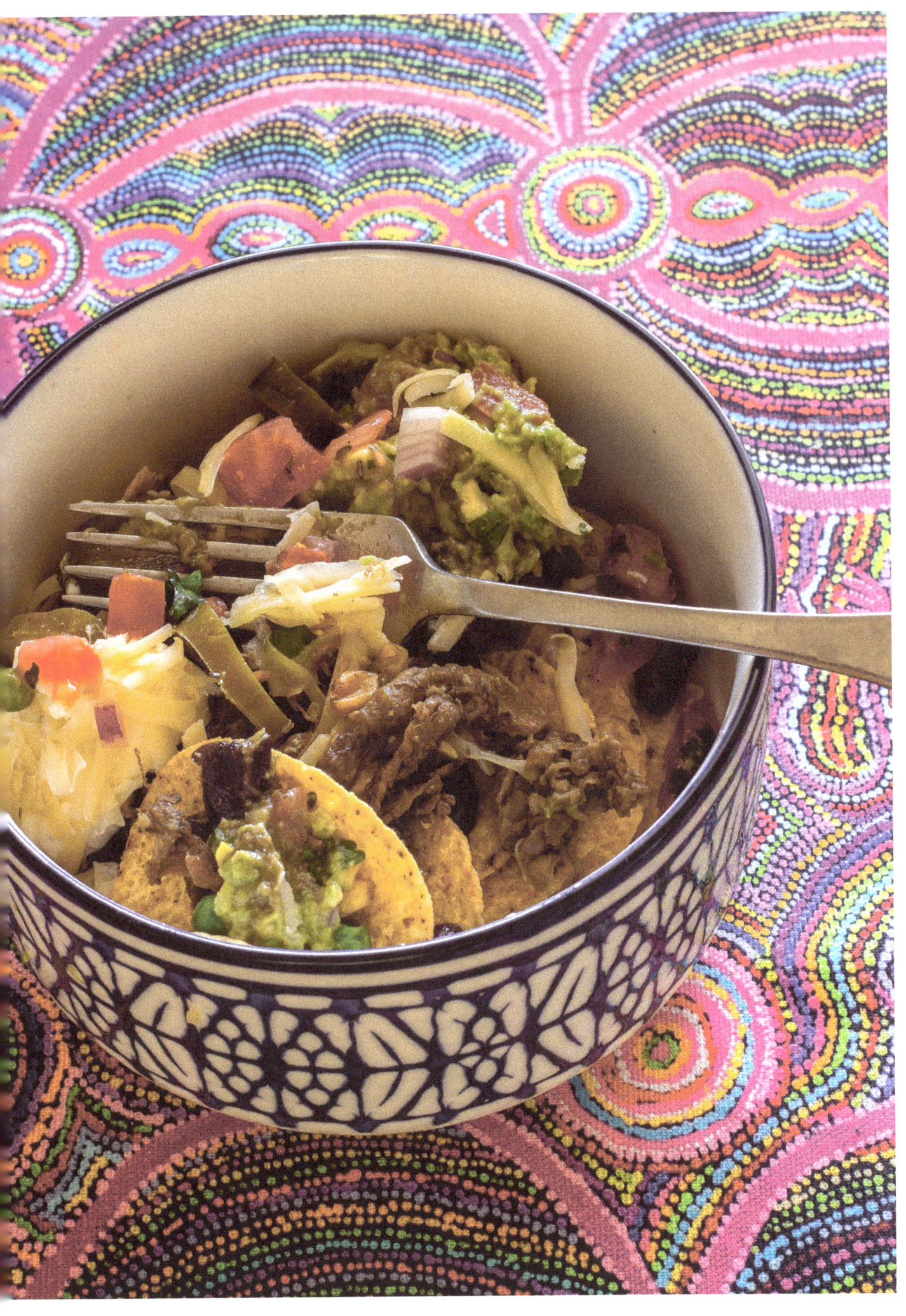

Mediterranean Pasta Salad

SERVES 4

This is a meal on its own but you can add in some spicy salami, chicken or serve it on the side of a steak or fish!

If you want to make your own pasta theres plenty of home made pasta recipes on my website or in my other cookbooks. Otherwise, use a good quality high protein pasta or for a gluten free version, use your favourite gluten free pasta. If we need more vegetables I will sometimes use one of the excellent wheat free vegetable pastas we can buy now. While going to the effort of preparing the vegetables, why not make extra for a vegetable lasagne (page 140) or the beautiful simple toasted paninis (page 70) to cook in the sandwich press at the office or workplace?

3 cups pasta (250g dry pasta)

1 cup beans

4 cups spinach or lettuce

½ cup sundried or fresh tomatoes

80 grams fetta

½ cup olives

1 large red capsicum

1 large zucchini

1 small eggplant

2 cups mushrooms

1 teaspoon basil (more if fresh leaves)

1 teaspoon oregano

1 clove of garlic

1 tablespoon balsamic

2 tablespoons robust extra virgin olive oil

Heat the oven to 180°C.

Cook the pasta to the packet instructions. Slice the eggplant into 1cm slices and rub salt into flesh and leave for around ½ hour, this will remove some bitterness. Rinse well and coat in oil and place on a baking tray. Slice zucchini, coat with oil and place on a baking tray. Wash and slice mushrooms and coat in oil and place on the baking tray. Roast the zucchini, mushrooms and eggplant for around 15 minutes or until cooked through. Roast the capsicum by coating it in oil and placing in an oven tray and baking for around 15 minutes until the skin is crisp or burnt. Cool and peel of skin and discard seeds. To make the dressing, crush the garlic and chop the herbs if using fresh and mix well with the oil and vinegar. Toss altogether and serve.

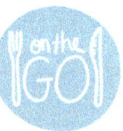

Do not add the spinach in. Dress your salad and put it in containers and then put the spinach in a pile on top to mix through just before eating. Store it for the whole day on ice in a cooler bag.

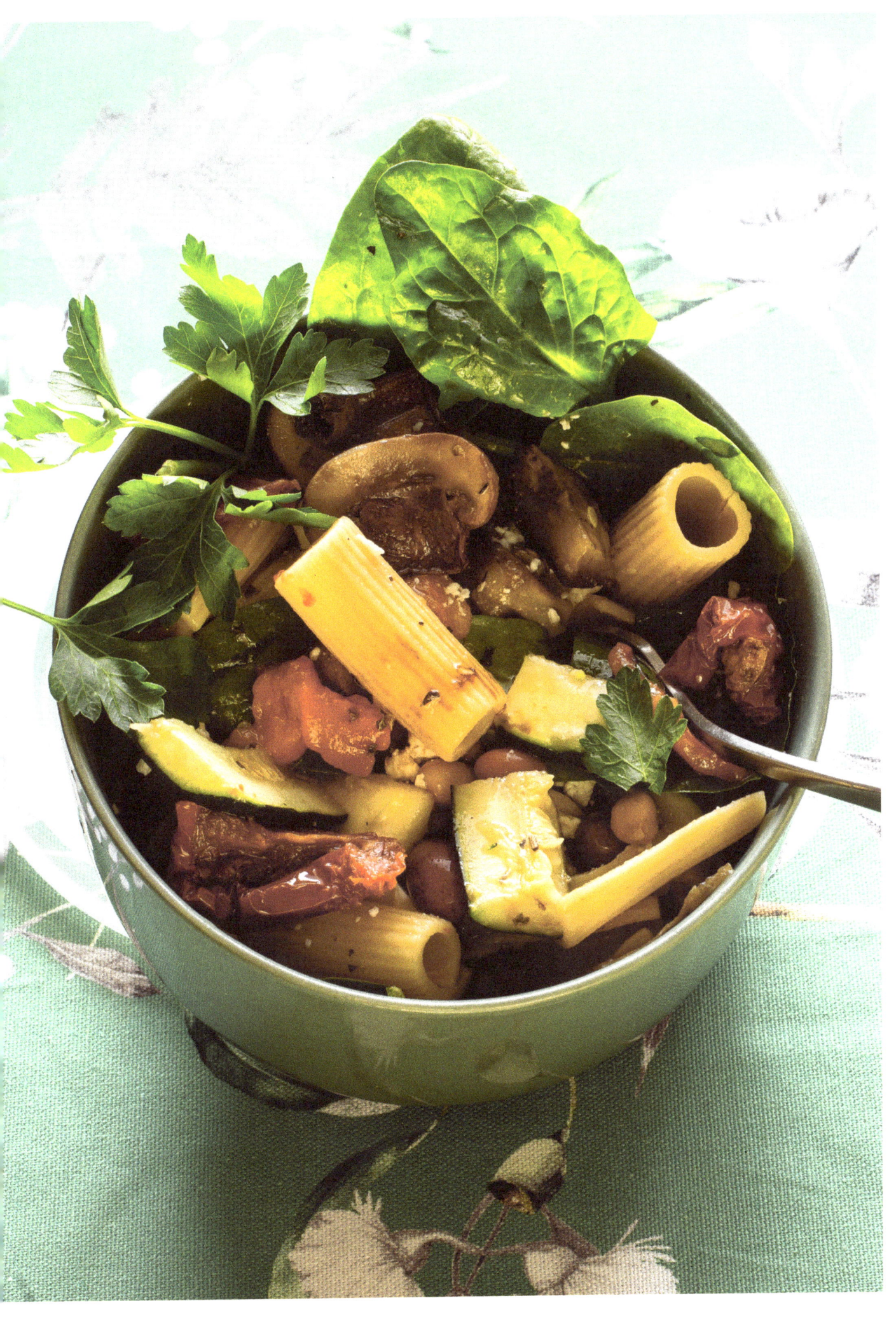

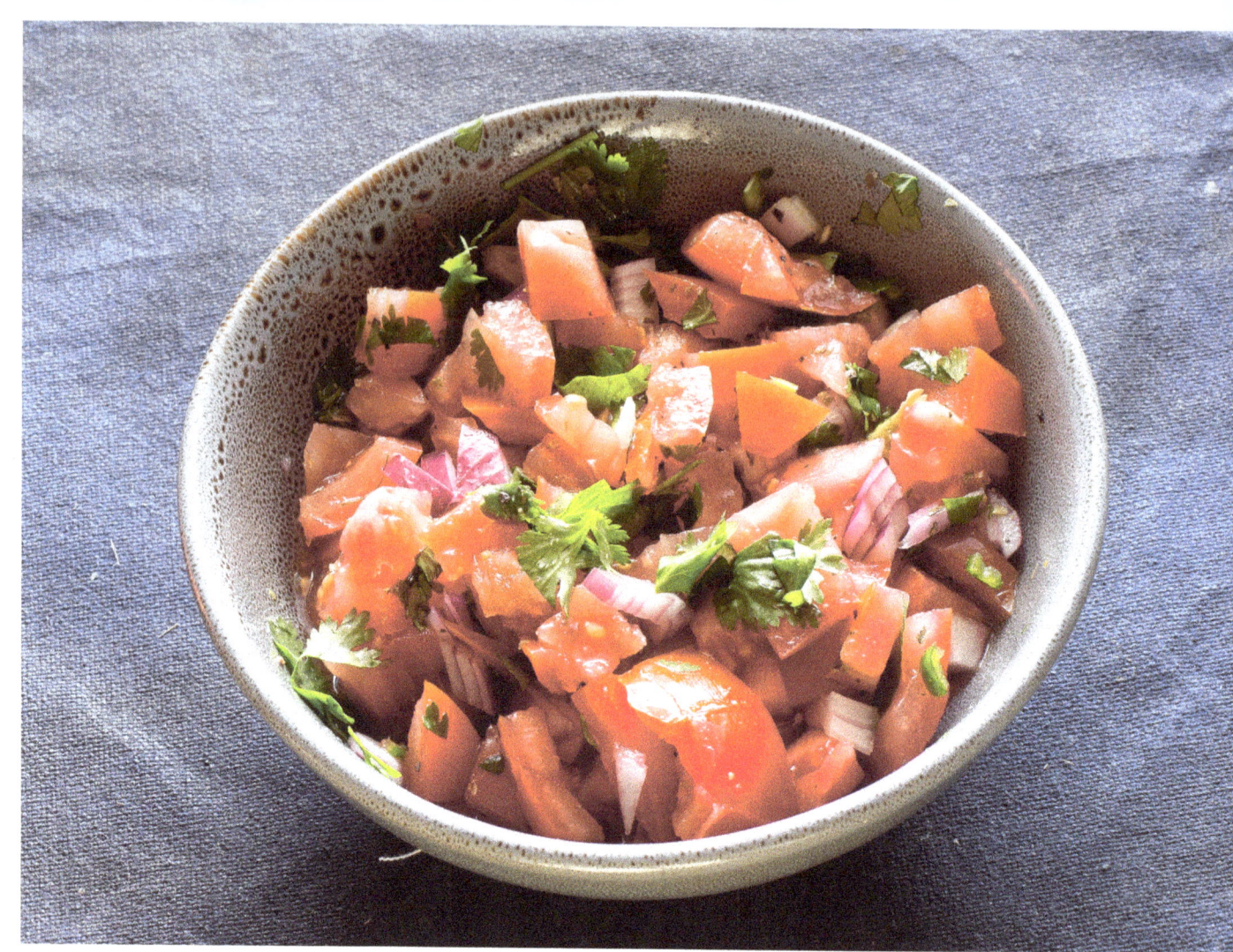

Fresh Salsa

MAKES A SIDE DISH

Best made in summer when there is a constant supply of tomatoes ripening on the bench and then served on everything from breakfast bruschetta's, salads, nachos, burgers and more.

2 large ripe tomatoes

1 tablespoon red onion

½ green chilli

1 tablespoon lime juice

2 tablespoons fresh coriander

pinch dried oregano

pinch dried chilli

salt to season

If you want to be posh you can remove the pulp and even skin, by blanching, from the tomato. But in the home kitchen I simply chop them in to a 5mm dice not to waste anything. Finely dice the onion and pepper and chop the coriander and mix well altogether with the oregano and chilli.

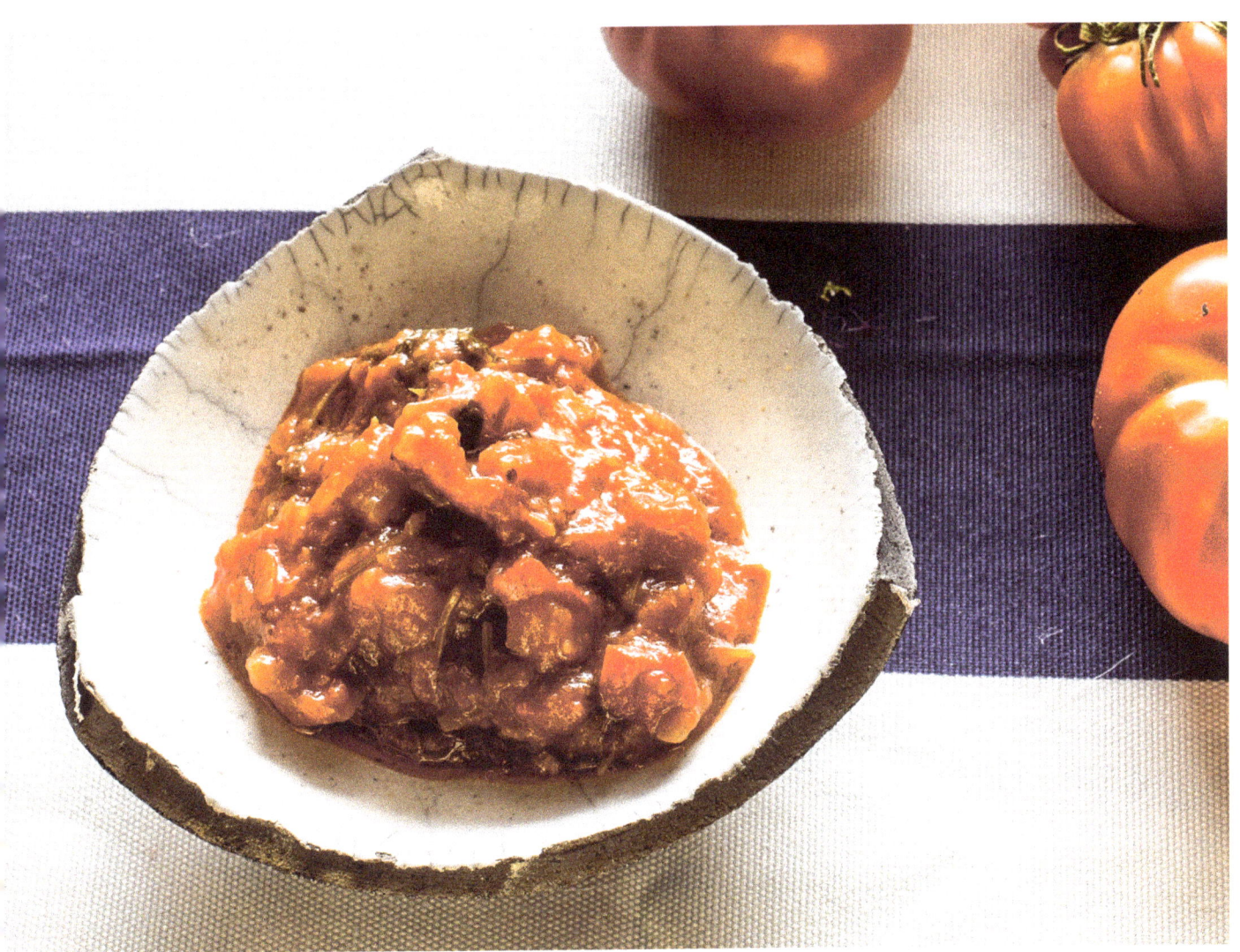

Cooked Salsa

MAKES ONE LARGE JAR

This salsa is a handy option for those winter months when you have preserved tomatoes to use and a tin works fine too.

1 green chilli

1 tablespoon robust extra virgin olive oil

1 red onion

1 garlic clove

400 grams crushed tomatoes

½ teaspoon salt

½ teaspoon cumin

½ teaspoon smoked paprika

½ teaspoon cinnamon

1 teaspoon dry oregano

4 sprigs coriander

Finely dice the chilli, onion, garlic and sauté in a heavy based pot with the extra virgin olive oil, salt, cumin, paprika, cinnamon and oregano over a medium heat. Add the tomato and continue simmering for around 20 minutes. Add coriander and just cook though. Serve hot or cold.

Corn Salad

MAKES FAMILY SIZE SIDE

The corn is best taken from a cob roasted in the husk with a dash of extra virgin olive oil and sea salt, but a can of corn or some frozen corn when not in the summer growing season. This is delicious packed with a piece of baked salmon cooled, smoked salmon, chicken or chunks of leftover roasted meats.

2 cups cooked black beans

2 cups corn kernels

½ red onion

2 large tomatoes

½ large cucumber

4 cups lettuce

¼ bunch fresh coriander

DRESSING

2 tablespoons extra virgin olive oil

1 tablespoon lime juice

1 tablespoon lemon juice

1 clove garlic

½ teaspoon cumin

pepper

salt

Chop the tomato and cucumber into about a 5mm dice. Finely dice the red onion and chop the lettuce and coriander and toss with the corn and beans and dress just before serving.

To make the dressing crush the garlic and mix together well with the oil, juice and cumin and season well with the pepper and salt.

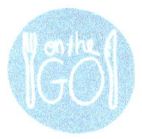

Leave the lettuce and coriander out when dressing the salad and sit them on top and mix through just before eating.

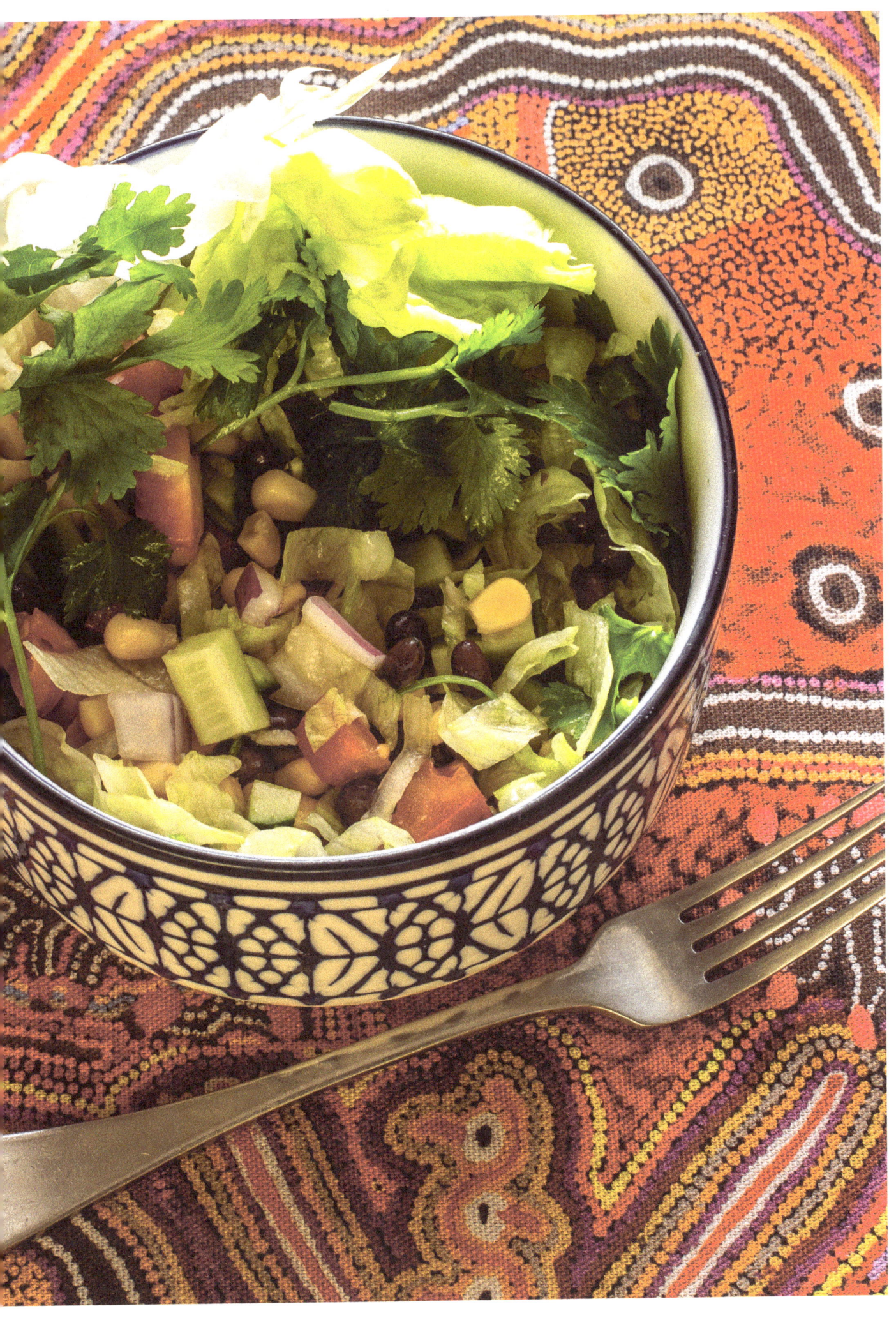

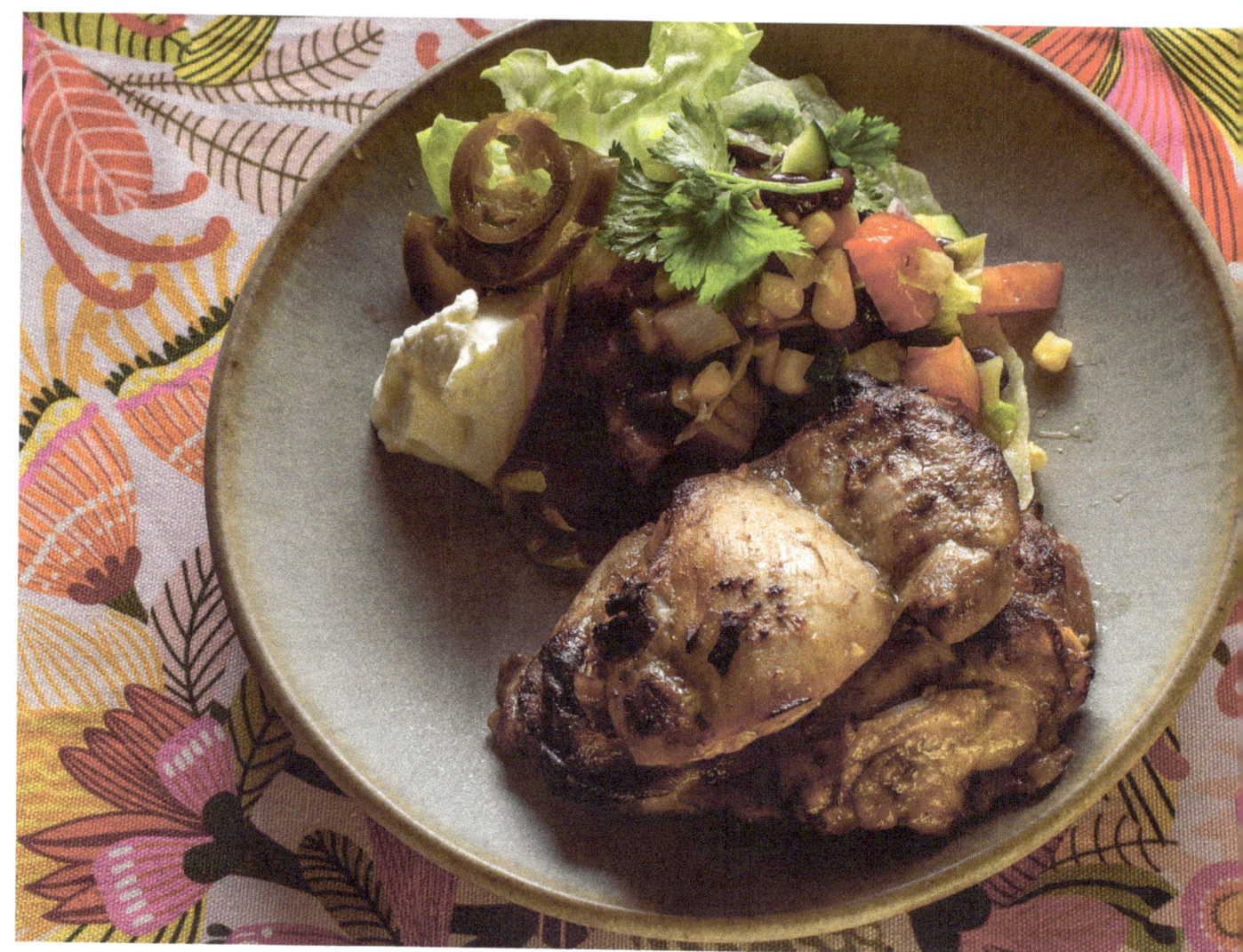

Honey Lime Chicken

SERVES 4-6

- 2 tablespoons honey
- 2 tablespoons lime
- 3 cloves garlic
- 1 teaspoon cumin
- ½ teaspoon cinnamon
- pinch white pepper
- ½ teaspoon coriander
- 1 teaspoon chilli
- 600 grams chicken thighs

Crush the garlic and mix well with all the other ingredients. Add the thighs, mix well and marinate overnight.

Heat the oven to 180°C.

Lay the thighs on a baking tray in a single layer and bake in the oven for around 20 minutes or until they are cooked through.

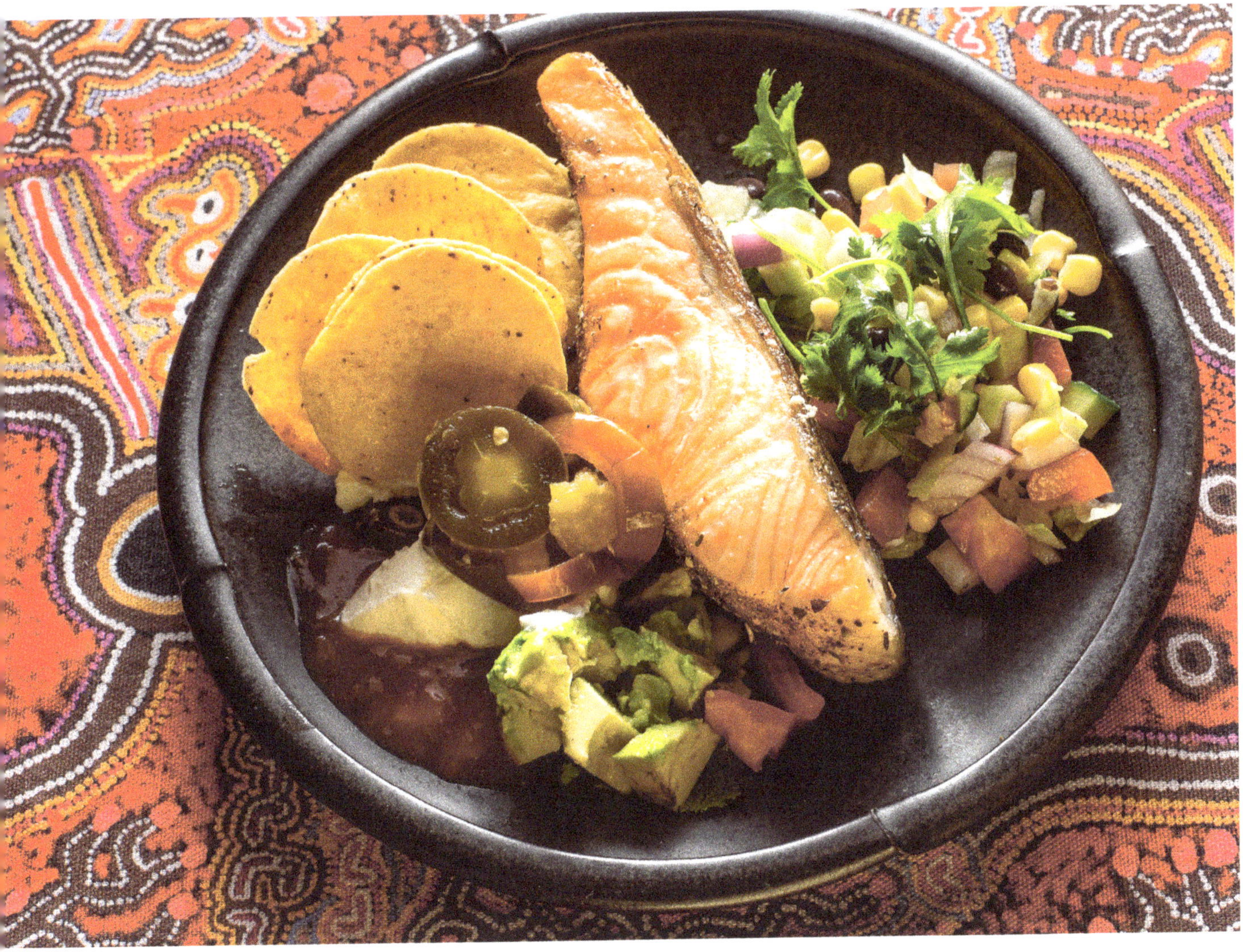

Spiced Tassal Salmon

SERVES 4

- 4 Tassal salmon steaks
- ½ teaspoon cumin
- ½ teaspoon coriander
- ½ teaspoon cinnamon
- ½ teaspoon cracked pepper
- ½ teaspoon sea salt
- 1 teaspoon oregano
- 1 teaspoon smoked paprika
- ¼ teaspoon dry chilli
- 1 tablespoon extra-virgin olive oil

Mix all the spices together well and coat the salmon.

Heat the oven to 160°C.

Heat the oil in an oven proof pan over a medium heat and add the salmon and cook skin side down for a few minutes to create a crispy skin. Transfer the pan to the oven and cook for around 20 minutes at the low temperature until the fish is just set.

Serve immediately with a corn salad or leave to cool to pack and enjoy cold.

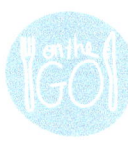

The oil content of salmon makes it's a delicious option to enjoy cold.

Chilli Con Carne

SERVES 4-6

We buy our beef by the side direct from the farmers so we always have plenty of beef mince. We are lucky the kids love this chilli con carne that can go on nachos, tacos, burritos, on baked spuds or simply with rice. I always have some in the freezer for a quick meal to pull together.

2 tablespoons extra virgin olive oil

1 teaspoon cinnamon

2 teaspoons cumin

½ teaspoon cracked black pepper

1 teaspoon oregano

½ teaspoon dry chilli flakes

500 grams beef mince

2 onions

1 red capsicum

1 carrot

4 cloves garlic

1 stick celery

400 grams tomatoes

½ teaspoon sea salt

TO SERVE

2 cups cooked red kidney beans

1 cup corn kernels

Finely dice the onion and crush the garlic. In a large heavy based pot heat the oil and add the cinnamon, cumin, pepper, chilli, onion, garlic, and oregano sauté until soft and fragrant for a minute or two.

Add mince and cook until browned. Add chopped capsicum, celery, carrot and tomatoes and lower the temperature and simmer for around 30 minutes until all cooked through. Season with the salt and add the beans and corn just before serving.

Freezer Tip: I will make this in bulk and freeze WITHOUT the beans and corn I will add them when re-heating.

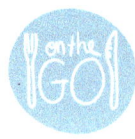

Pop the hot chilli con carne in a thermos and pack corn chips in a container and sauces such as salsa and sour cream in a separate containers to plonk on top on corn chips when ready to eat. There are better brand corn chips fewer ingredients on the label are generally better for us.

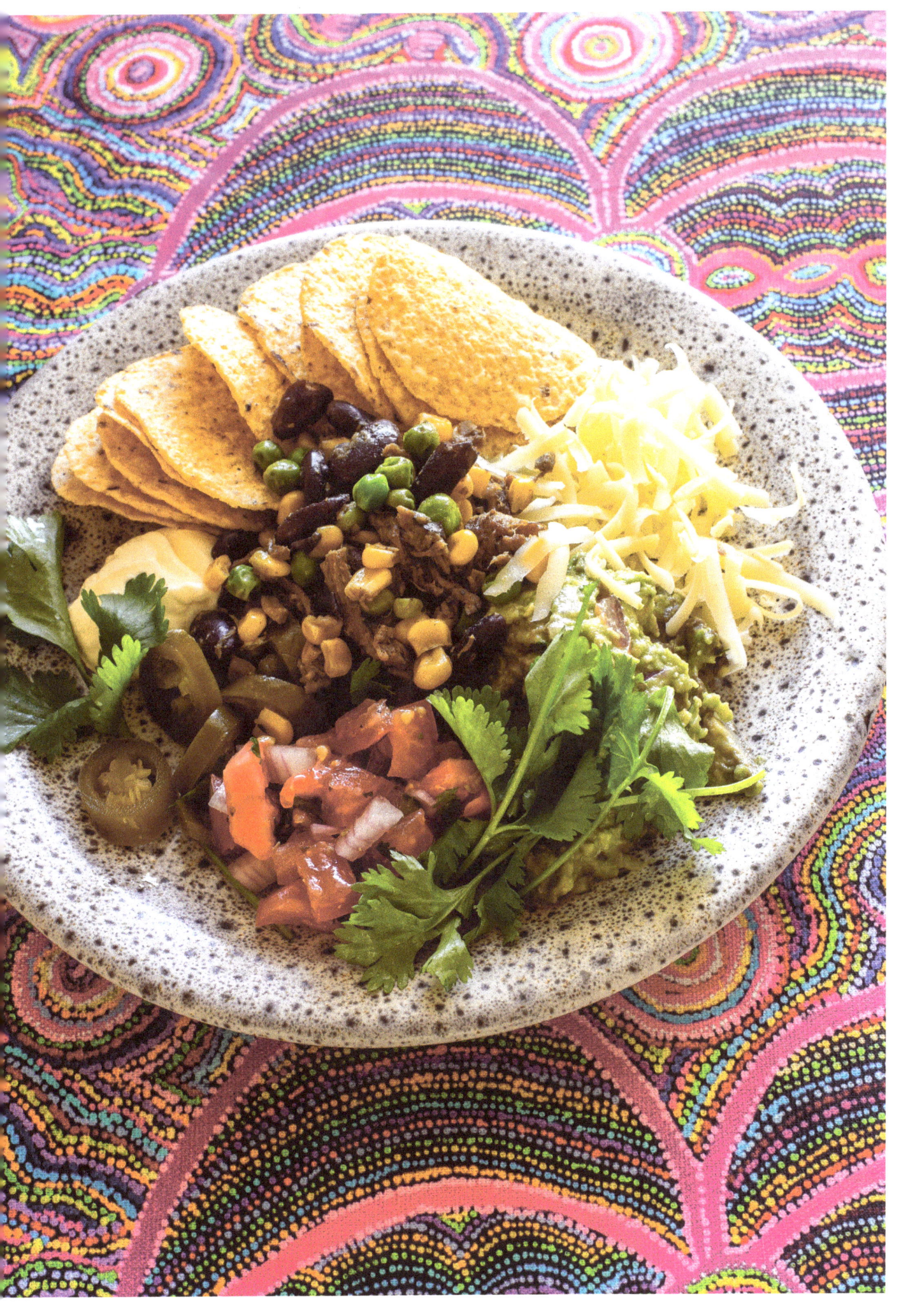

Guacamole

MAKES ENOUGH FOR A FAMILY SIDE DISH

Add chilli for a spicy dip, but if you are serving your guacamole on the side of something spicy then you may want to keep it cool to contrast the heat so leave the chilli out.

4 small avocados

1 tablespoon red onion

1 tablespoon coriander

pinch cumin

pinch oregano

pinch seas salt

pinch pepper

½ tomatoes

1 tablespoon lime juice

Green chilli (optional)

Remove the skin and pip from the avocado and dice. Chop the onion into a fine dice and add to the avocado with the chopped coriander, cumin, oregano, salt, pepper, and finely diced tomato, lime juice and chilli if you are using. Mix well and serve.

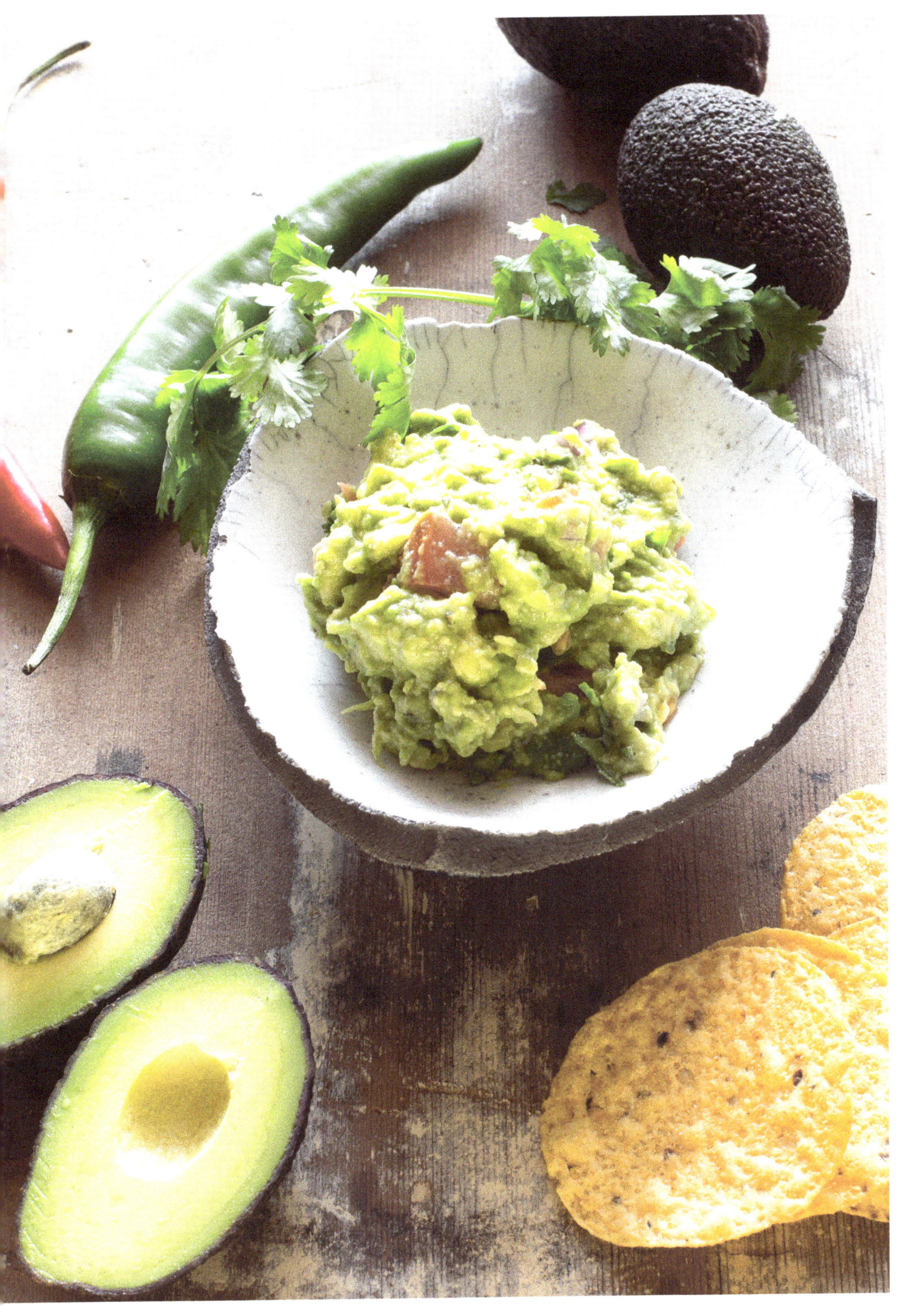

Honey and Soy Chicken Nori Rolls

SERVES 6

There are loads of ideas for different fillings for nori rolls. Leftover roast chicken or plain grilled or steamed chicken, salmon, tuna, avocado, egg tofu and more. I put the rice on thin so I can get ½ to one cup plus a good portion of protein in each roll. Some sushi from the shop you are really just buying nutrient lacking rice!

1 cup sushi rice

1 tablespoon rice wine vinegar

1 teaspoon caster sugar

6 nori sheets

2 tablespoons mayonnaise (see page 25)

FILLING

4 chicken thigh schnitzels (page 34)

2 carrots

1 cucumber

½ capsicum

½ cup bean sprouts

2 spring onions

To cook the rice, place the rice in a colander and rinse under cold running water for a minute to wash off any excess starch. Put the rice into a heavy based saucepan with 1 ½ cups water. Bring to a gentle boil, reduce the heat and cook covered for about 12 minutes or until all of the water has been absorbed. Remove from the heat and leave to sit for 10 minutes covered to finish cooking. Add the vinegar and sugar to the rice and fold through and cool.

Lay the nori sheets on the bench and cover ¾ of each sheet with a thin layer of rice. Add grated carrot and strips of cucumber, capsicum, sprouts and spring onions, and slices of chicken and roll up with the empty part of the nori on the outside.

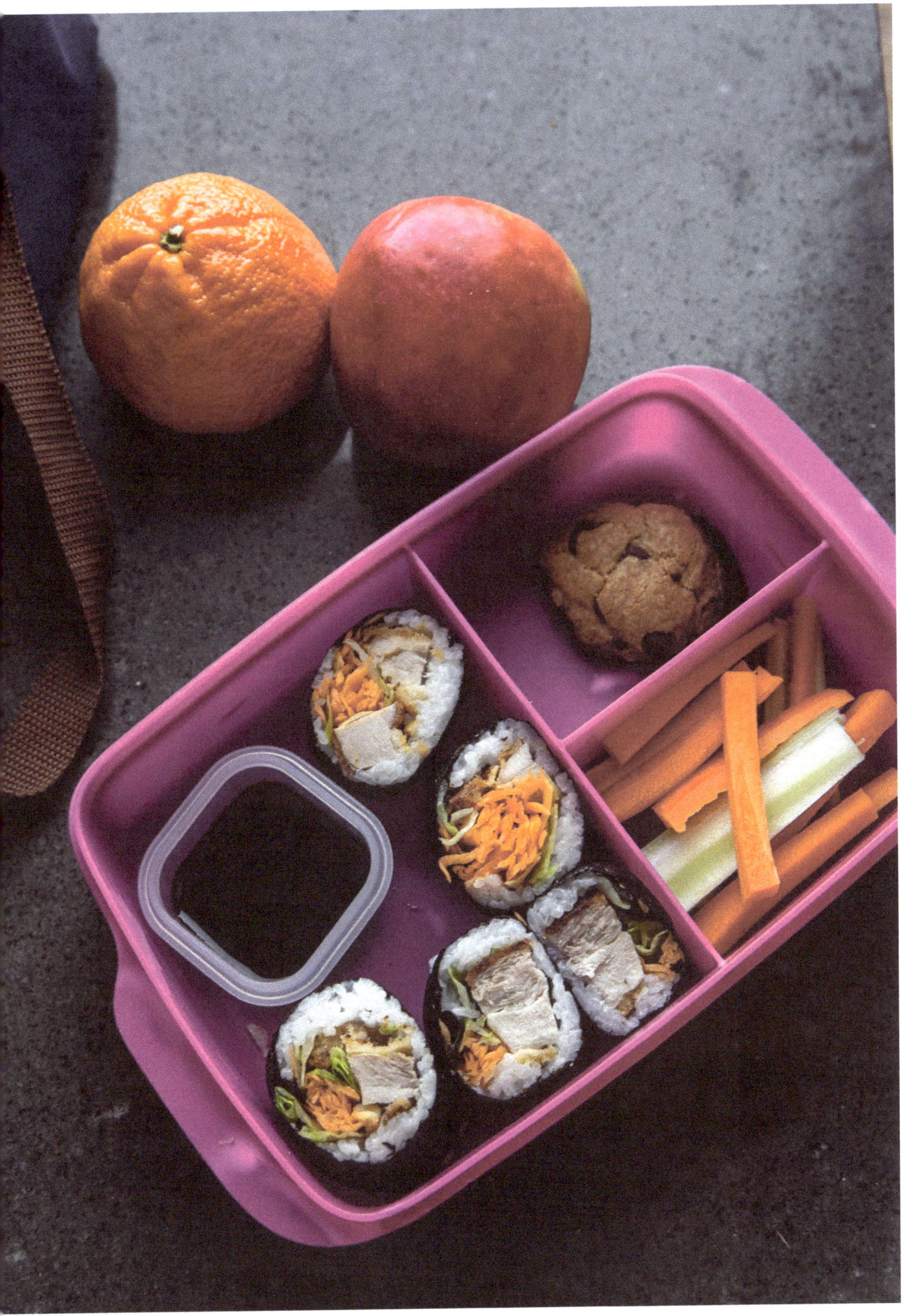

Honey and Cinnamon Nut Bar

MAKES 16

Try other seeds and nuts in these delicious bars, perfect for an after school before cricket or dancing snack.

50ml extra virgin olive oil

70 grams butter

3 tablespoons honey

1 ½ cups rolled oats

½ cup self-raising flour

2 teaspoons cinnamon

1 cup almonds

½ cup cacao buds

½ cup dates

½ cup hemp seeds

Heat the oven to 180°C.

Measure the butter, oil and honey, add to a saucepan and then melt over a low heat. Measure the other ingredients, place in a bowl and beat well to combine. Line a 20cm square cake tin with baking paper.

Spoon the mixture into the baking dish, bake for approximately

25 minutes or until golden brown and cooked through.

Cool. Cut into bars.

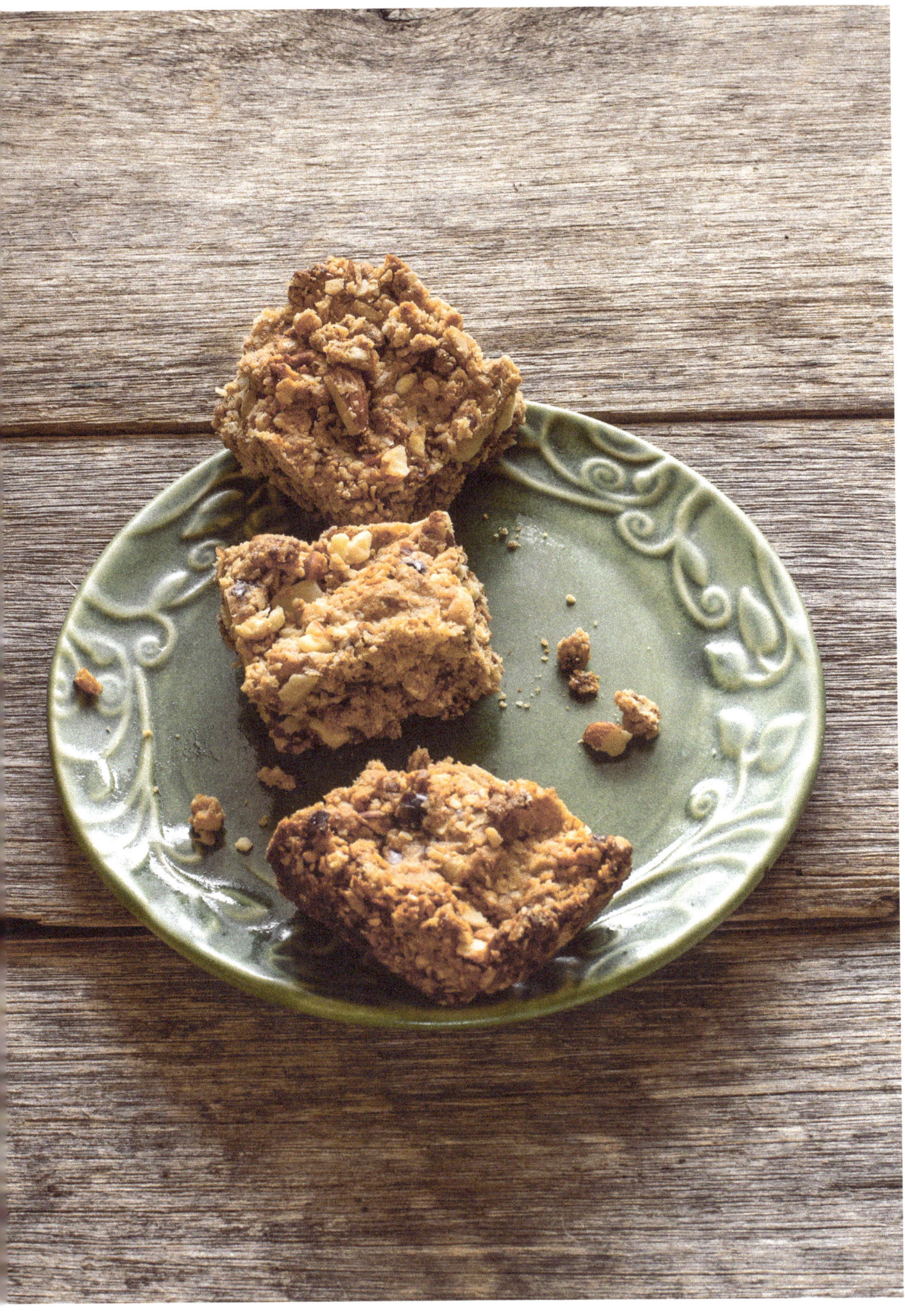

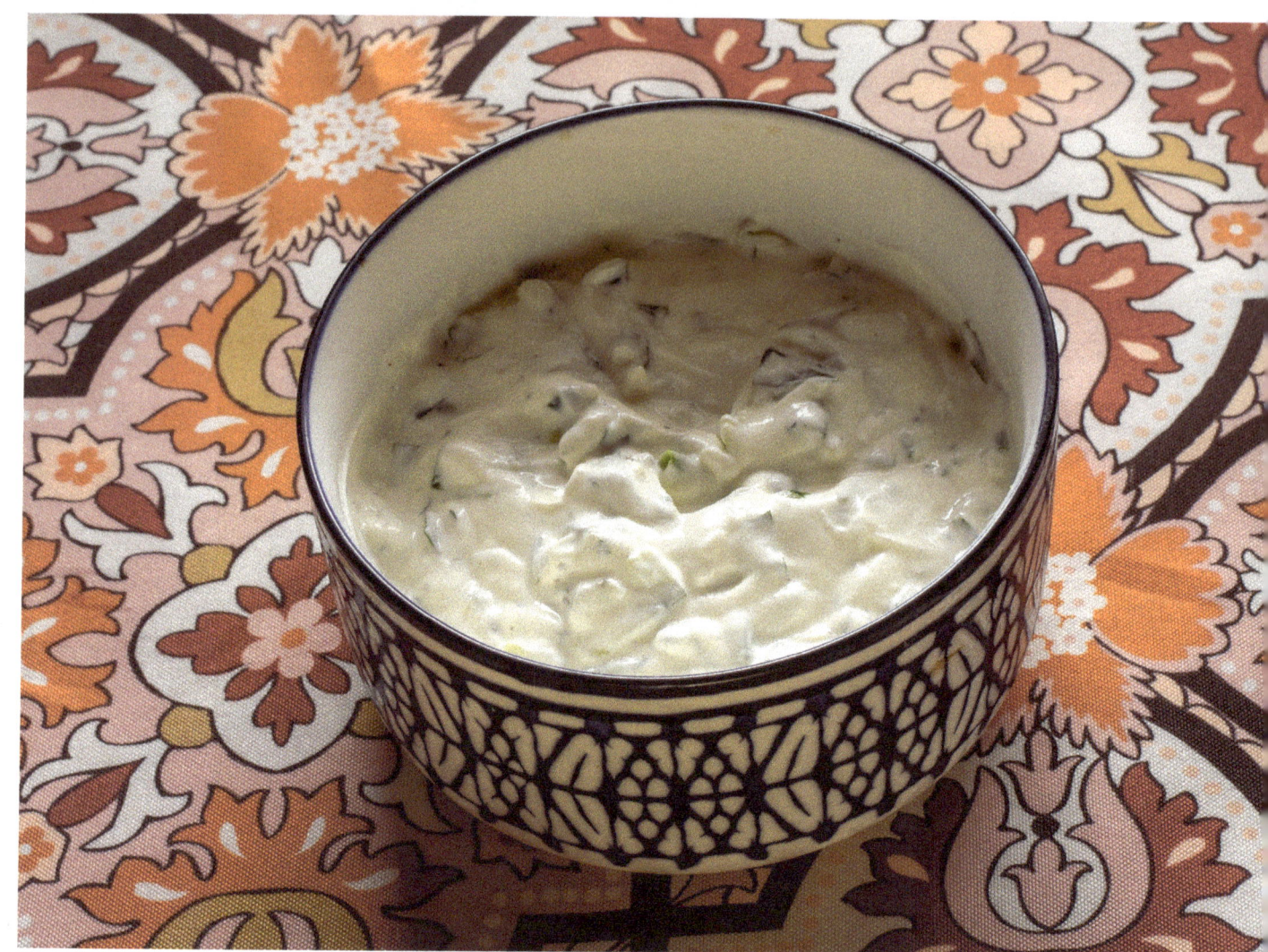

Tzatziki Dip

MAKES A SMALL CONTAINER

1 cup natural yogurt
half large cucumber
1 tablespoon dill
2 cloves garlic
salt and pepper
¼ teaspoon cumin

Cut the cucumber in half, scoop out the seeds and dice into a small dice. Crush the garlic and mix with the yogurt, cucumber chopped dill, cumin and then season with salt and pepper.

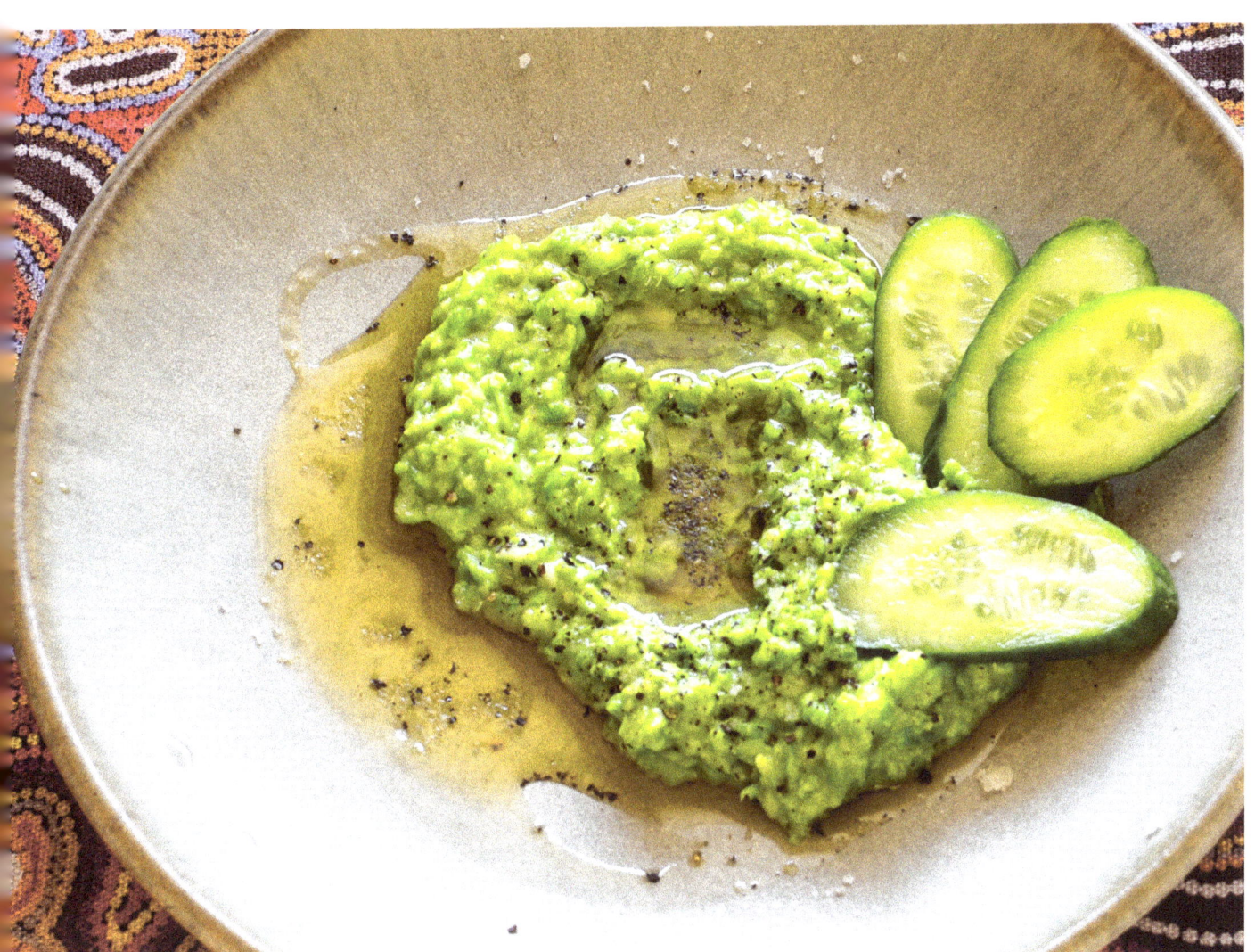

Pea Hummus

MAKES A SMALL JAR

For a quick addition of a green vegetable to the meal or day this pea hummus made with frozen peas is a handy choice. You can also use soaked or tinned chickpeas, white beans or roasted veggies like pumpkin or sweet potato.

200 grams green peas

5 cloves garlic

robust extra virgin olive oil (approx 100ml)

juice of 2 lemons

sea salt

pepper

In the thermocooker or blender blend all the ingredients together to form a smooth paste.

Season well with salt and pepper.

Slow Cooked Mediterranean Lamb Shoulder

MAKES ENOUGH FOR A FEW FAMILY MEALS

This meat makes an amazing souvlaki with tzatziki (page 60), wraps (page 66) and salad.

I use the slow cooker but you could use a low oven with the meat in a lidded oven proof dish. Just remember all bench top slow cookers will cook at different times so get to know your own.

approximately 2 kilos lamb shoulder

MARINADE

2 tablespoons extra virgin olive oil

6 cloves garlic

1 brown onion

1 sprig rosemary

4 sage leaves

2 teaspoons dry oregano

1 teaspoon dry basil

½ teaspoon pepper

1 teaspoon smoked paprika

1 teaspoon dry parsley

Peel the garlic and onion and place in the thermocooker or food processor with all the marinade ingredients and blend until you make a smooth paste. Rub all over meat and pop in a lidded container and marinate in the fringe at least overnight.

Place the meat in the slow cooker and cook on high for around 5 hours or until you can pull all the meat apart with forks.

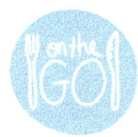

Pack the meat in a container that keeps food hot and the salad, wrap and sauce in cool containers to put together a quick and healthy souvlaki on the go.

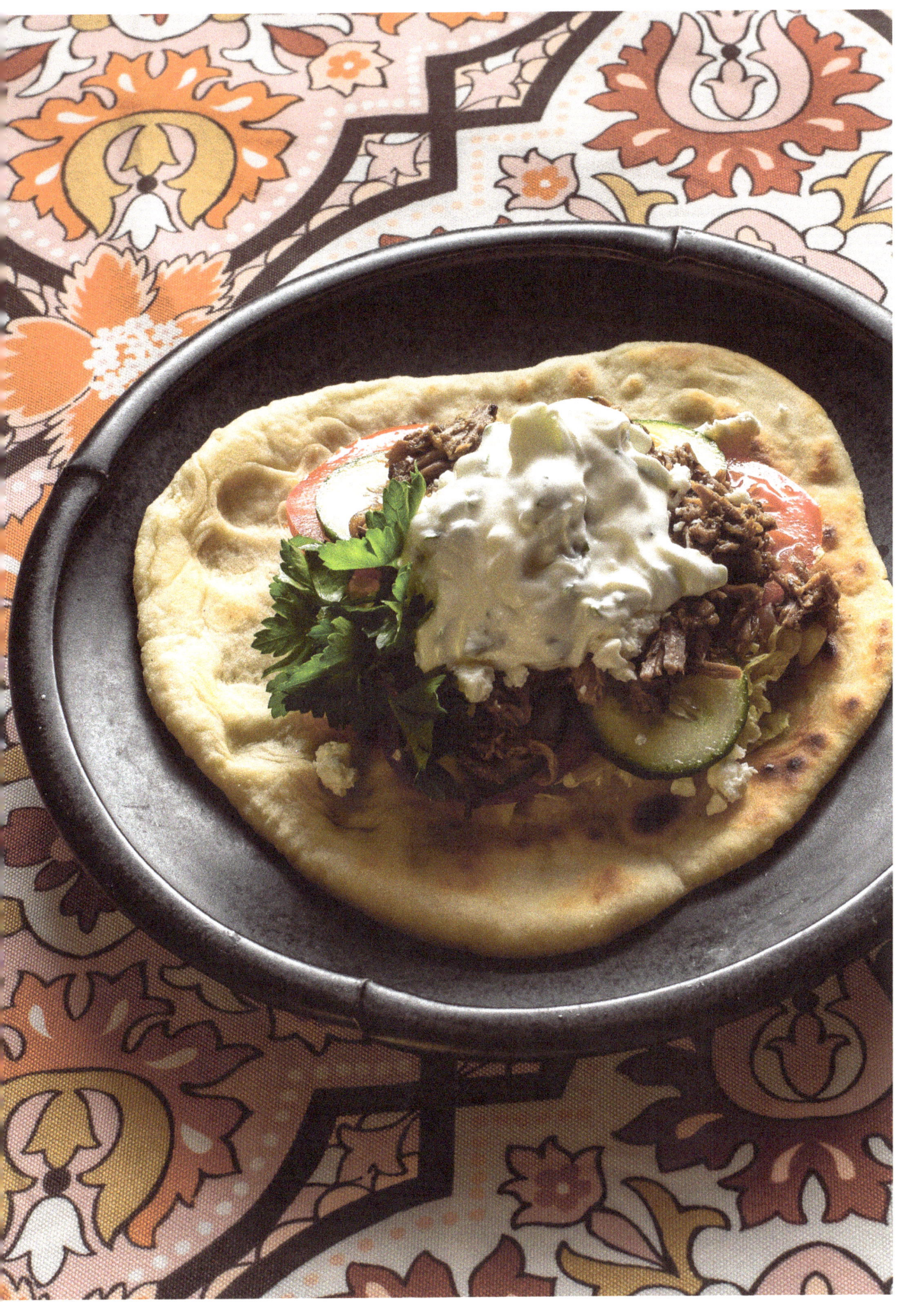

Savoury Rice Breakie Porridge

SERVES 2

Congee is a Chinese rice porridge style breakfast. I like it as it is a great way to get bone broth and veggies in for breakfast. It's a handy packed lunch or dinner too. There are all sorts of pickles, preserves and fermented things you can serve on top and all sorts of vegetable and meat combinations you can put in it. I always have brown rice cooked in broth on hand in my fridge or freezer. After I have made the broth I strain it and put it back in the same slow cooker to cook the rice. The meat is chicken I have pulled from the carcass when I make a stock but you can use left over roasted meats.

extra virgin olive oil

1 cup cooked brown rice (see page 29 basics)

2 cups chicken stock

1 cup chicken meat

1 cup mushrooms

½ cup corn kernels

½ cup cabbage

TO SERVE

dash soy sauce

chilli

spring onions

kimchi

In a small heavy based pot sauté the mushrooms and cabbage in a dash of extra virgin olive oil until soft. Add the stock, corn and rice and corn and a dash of soy sauce and cook through. Serve with fresh chopped chilli and spring onions and kimchi.

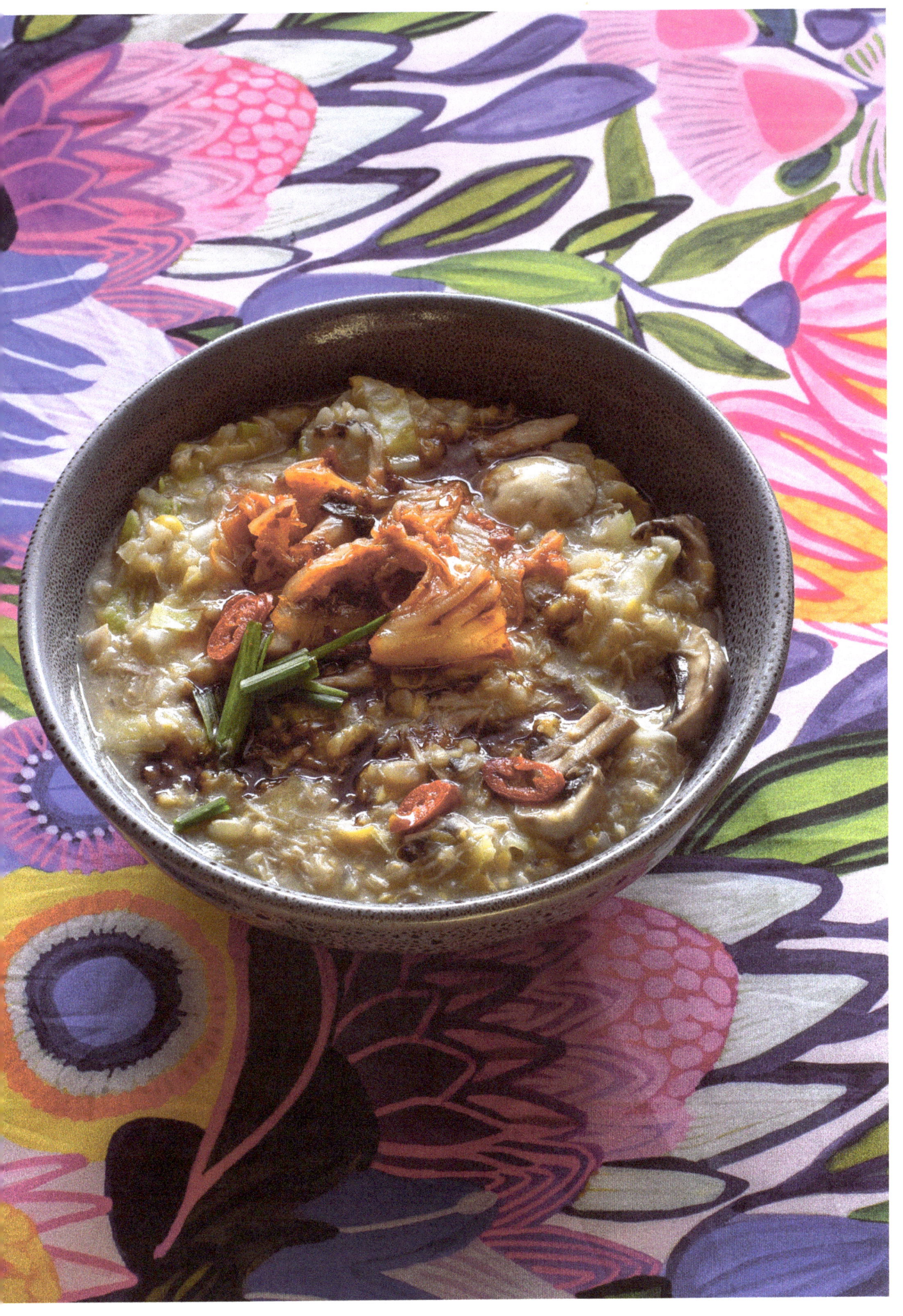

Wraps

MAKES 12

I find the commercial packets of wraps handy, but my kids will not eat them untoasted as there is a weird taste or smell to them. Must be the preservatives! Anyway you need to wonder why they last so long on the shelf? Yuck.

These wraps freeze well between layers of baking paper (reuse many times) and it's the thought of making them that seems massive, the mess, all the rolling and then the cooking BUT honestly once you start it tastes no time at all, the rolling as quite therapeutic and they really are delicious!!

400 grams self-raising flour

1 teaspoon salt

½ cup extra virgin olive oil

1 cup water

Mix all ingredients well together. Cut into 12 portions and roll into balls and rest.

Roll out each ball to fit and large 20 cm flat base frying pan. Over a medium heat with a spray of dash of extra virgin olive oil cook each wrap until golden brown.

Stack and store in a tea towel to keep warm.

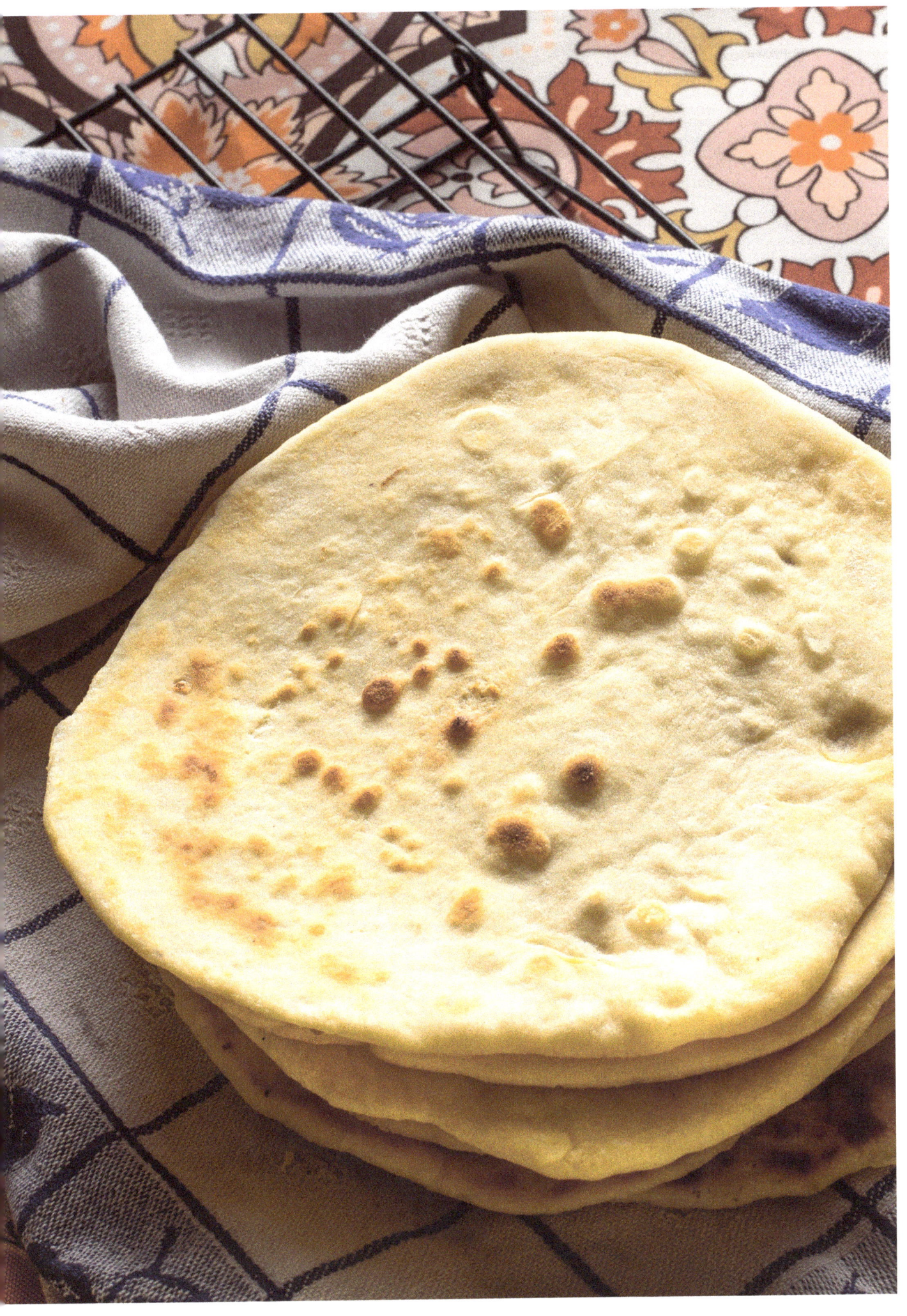

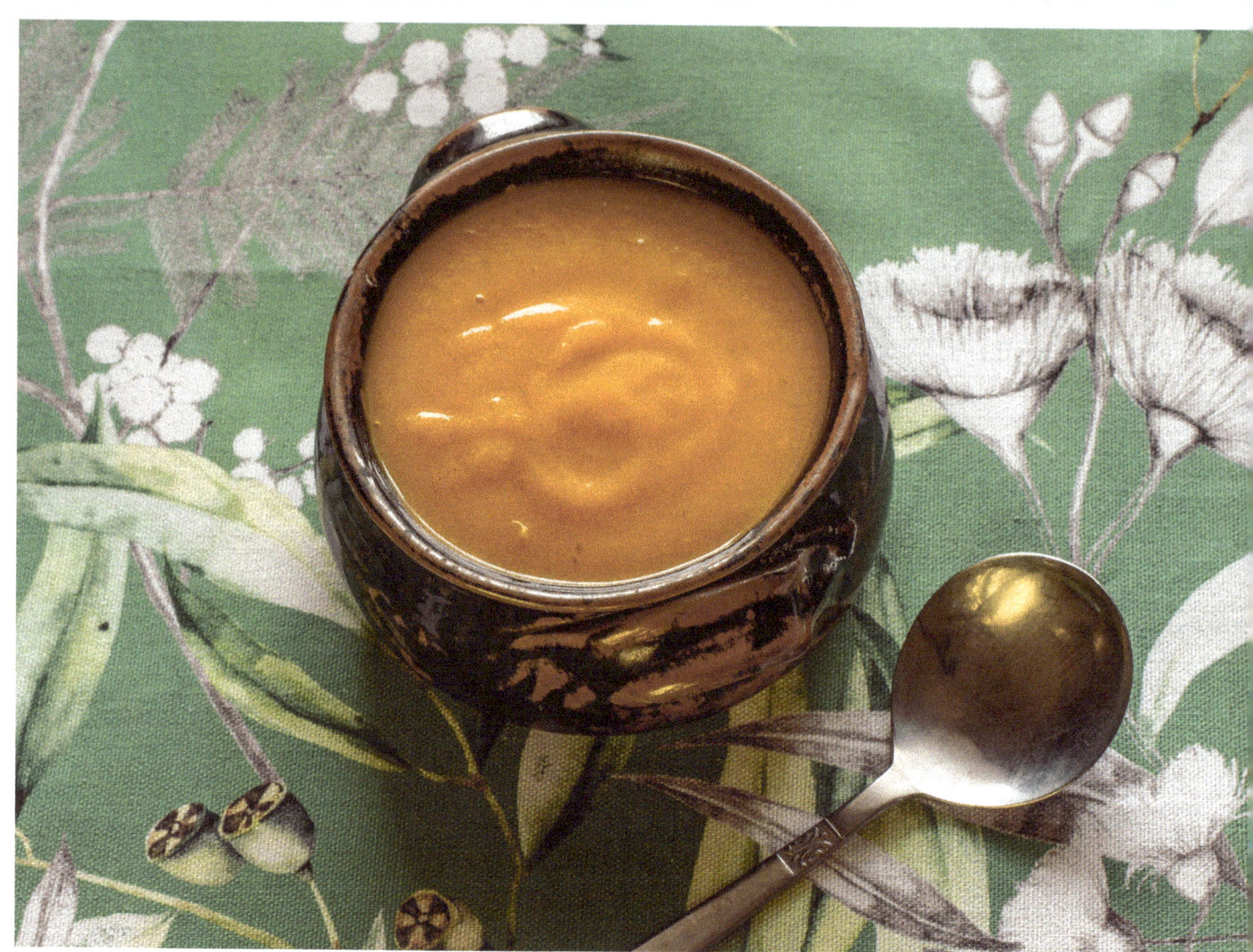

Carrot and Pumpkin Soup

SERVES 6

Soups are the easiest way to consume a few extra veggies! Easy to prepare they freeze well to simply heat and pop in the thermos to pack for lunch to go with a few boiled eggs or a tin of fish from the pantry.

1 tablespoon butter

2 cloves garlic

20 big sage leaves

5 large carrots

1 onion

1 litre chicken stock

300 grams pumpkin

pepper and salt

In a large heavy base pot heat the butter until it starts to froth and slightly brown add roughly chopped garlic and sage and sauté until tender. Add roughly chopped carrots and onion and sauté for a further 3 minutes and then add stock, pumpkin and a pinch of pepper and bring to the boil and simmer gently for about 20 minutes or until the carrots and pumpkin are cooked and soft. Puree in a blender or with a stick blender and season with salt and pepper and serve.

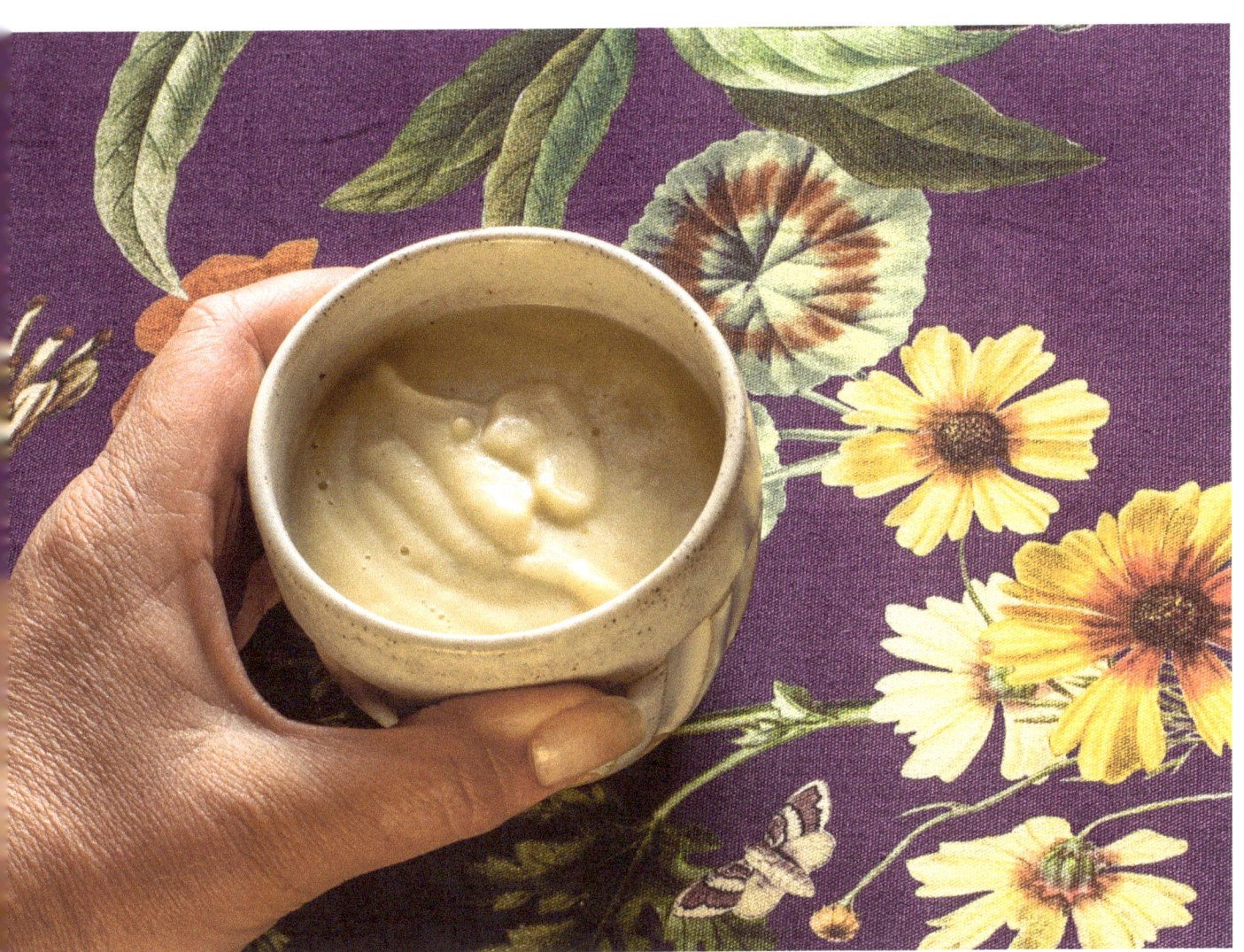

Cauliflower Soup

SERVES 4

Try adding a few tablespoons of cheese to this soup to make it a little fancier, a blue cheese or aged cheddar would work well.

1 cauliflower

1 brown onion

2 cloves garlic

500ml chicken stock

100ml cream

2 tablespoons tarragon

salt and pepper

Peel and dice garlic and onion and fry in the oil, add cauliflower and stock and bring to the boil and simmer for 15 minutes, add tarragon and cream and puree. Season with salt and pepper and serve

Grilled Mediterranean Vegetable Panini

SERVES 4

The ideas for these sandwiches are limitless. Different cheeses and meats, leftover roasts, tandoori chicken, mustards and pickles, roasted pumpkin or beetroot. Yum!

4 paninis or focaccias

4 cups spinach or lettuce

½ cup sundried or fresh tomatoes

80 grams fetta

½ cup olives

1 large red capsicum

1 large zucchini

1 small eggplant

2 cups mushrooms

Slice the eggplant into 1cm slices and rub salt into flesh and leave for around ½ hour this will remove some bitterness. Rinse well and coat in oil and place on a baking tray. Slice zucchini, coating with oil and place on a baking tray. Wash and slice mushrooms and coat in oil and place on the baking tray. Roast the zucchini, mushrooms and eggplant for around 15 minutes or until cooked through. Roast the capsicum by coating it in oil and placing in an oven tray and baking for around 15 minutes until the skin is crisp or burnt. Cool and peel off skin and discard seeds.

Cut the panini in half and fill with layers of the vegetables, fetta, olives and vegetables and toast in a sandwich press or bake in the oven.

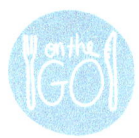

Prep your veggies on the weekend to prepare this beautiful panini or focaccia each morning to pop in the sandwich press at work. What would you pay for this in a fancy café?

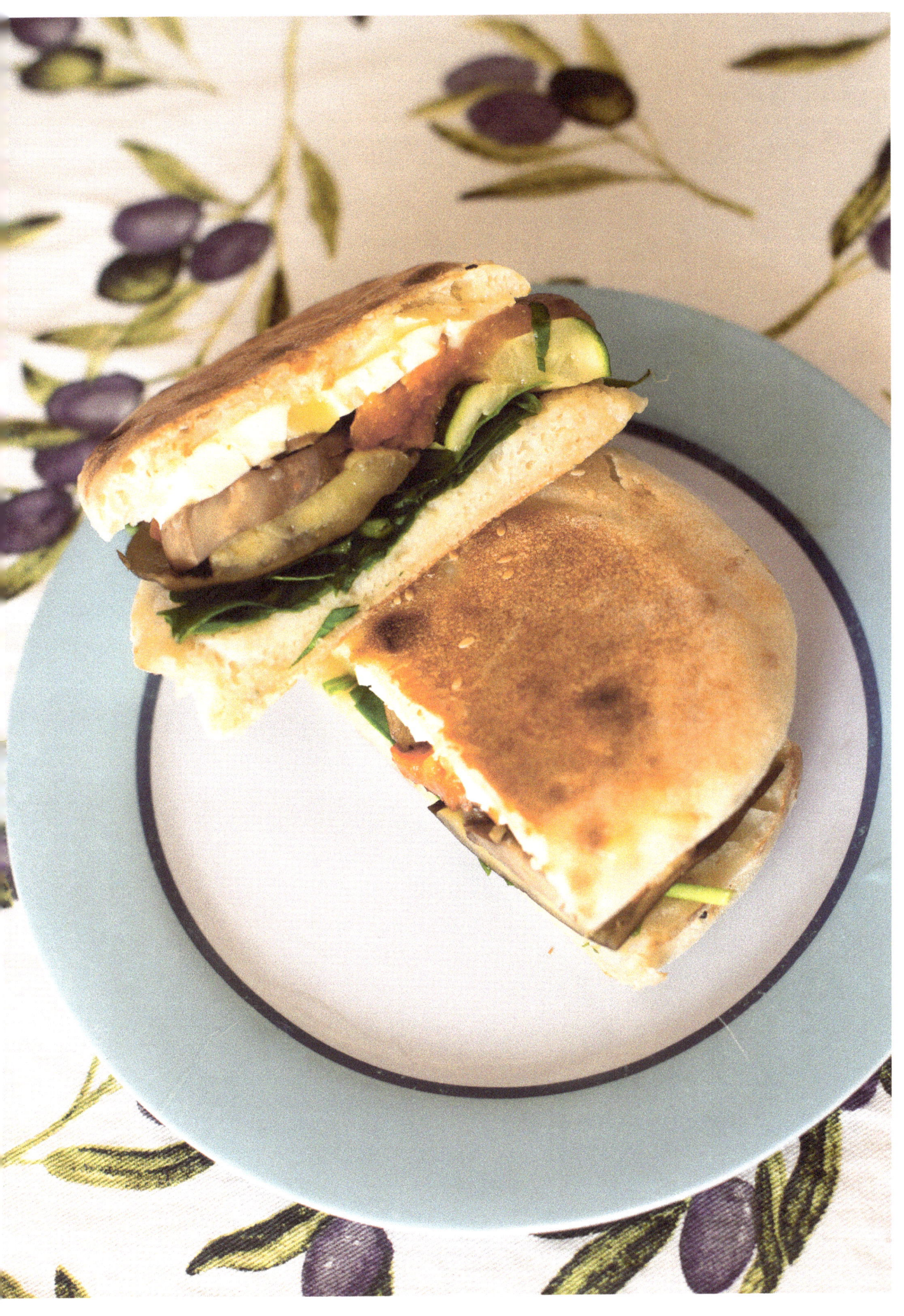

Mango Chicken

MAKES 2 FAMILY MEALS

2 tablespoons extra virgin olive oil

2 medium onions

½ red capsicum

3 cloves garlic

2cm knob ginger

½ teaspoon tumeric

½ teaspoon coriander

¼ teaspoon cayenne pepper

¼ teaspoon cinnamon

½ teaspoon ground fennel seed

¼ teaspoon black pepper

½ teaspoon cumin

2 mangoes

2 tablespoons apple cider vinegar

1 cup stock

1 cup coconut cream

1 kilo chicken thighs

salt and pepper

Finely dice the onion and crush the garlic and ginger, finely dice the capsicum. In a large heavy based pot heat the extra virgin olive oil and sauté the onion, garlic, ginger capsicum, spices until soft and fragrant. Add the mango, vinegar, coconut cream and simmer gently. Cut the chicken thighs into a 1cm dice, add and simmer gently until cooked through.

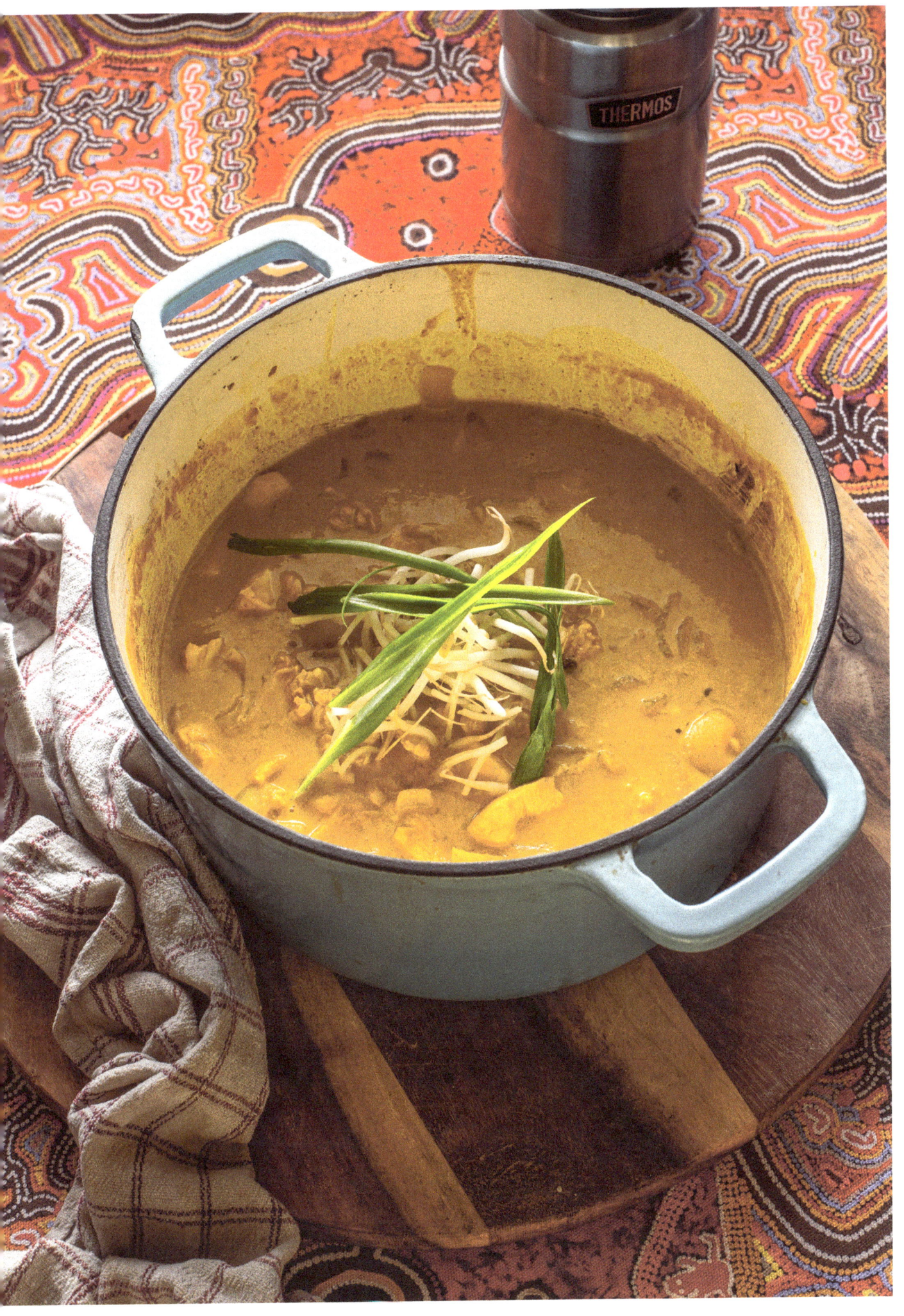

Spicy Pulled Pork

MAKES 3-4 FAMILY MEALS

Cook the 2 kilos and freeze a few extra portions for another day for family meals. Can be served with corn chips for loaded nachos, hard or soft tacos or in burritos or salads.

2 kilo pork shoulder

1 teaspoon salt

1 teaspoon black pepper

2 onions

1 large red chilli

6 cloves garlic

2 tablespoons dry oregano

2 teaspoons cumin

1 tablespoon extra virgin olive oil

1 teaspoon cinnamon

1 tablespoon smoked paprika

1 tablespoon honey

1 tablespoon lemon juice

1 tablespoon lime juices

Bring the pork to room temperature on the bench. Peel garlic and onion and pop in the thermocooker or food processor with all the other ingredients and blend until a chunky paste. Rub all over the pork and put in the slow cooker on high, or a covered dish in a low oven, for around 4 hours until the pork is tender and can be pulled apart with forks.

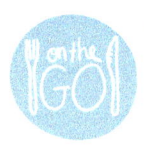 *Put the meat in a container that keeps food hot to dump on the corn chips and salads and dressings to eat on the go.*

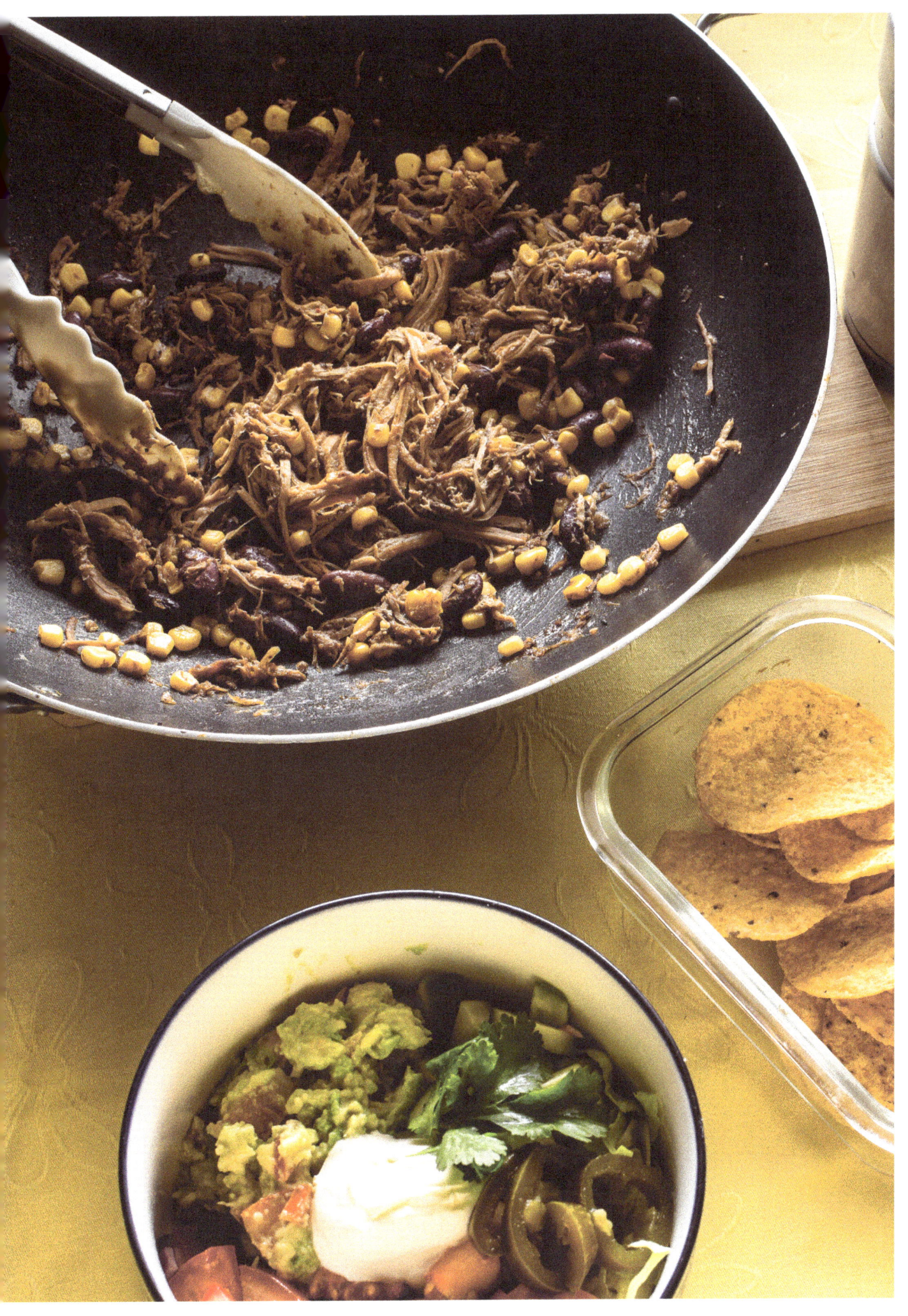

Lamb Kofta

SERVES 4-6

500 grams lamb mince

1 brown onion

2 garlic cloves

1 teaspoon cumin

1 teaspoon garam masala

1 teaspoon oregano

1 teaspoon smoked paprika

1 teaspoon parsley

Finely chop the onion and crush the garlic and mix well with the herbs and spices and mince. Wrap 2 tablespoon size handfuls of the meat mix around sticks. In a large pan over medium heat cook the koftas until cooked through.

Serve hot or cold with a dip like tzatziki (page 60)or hummus and salad.

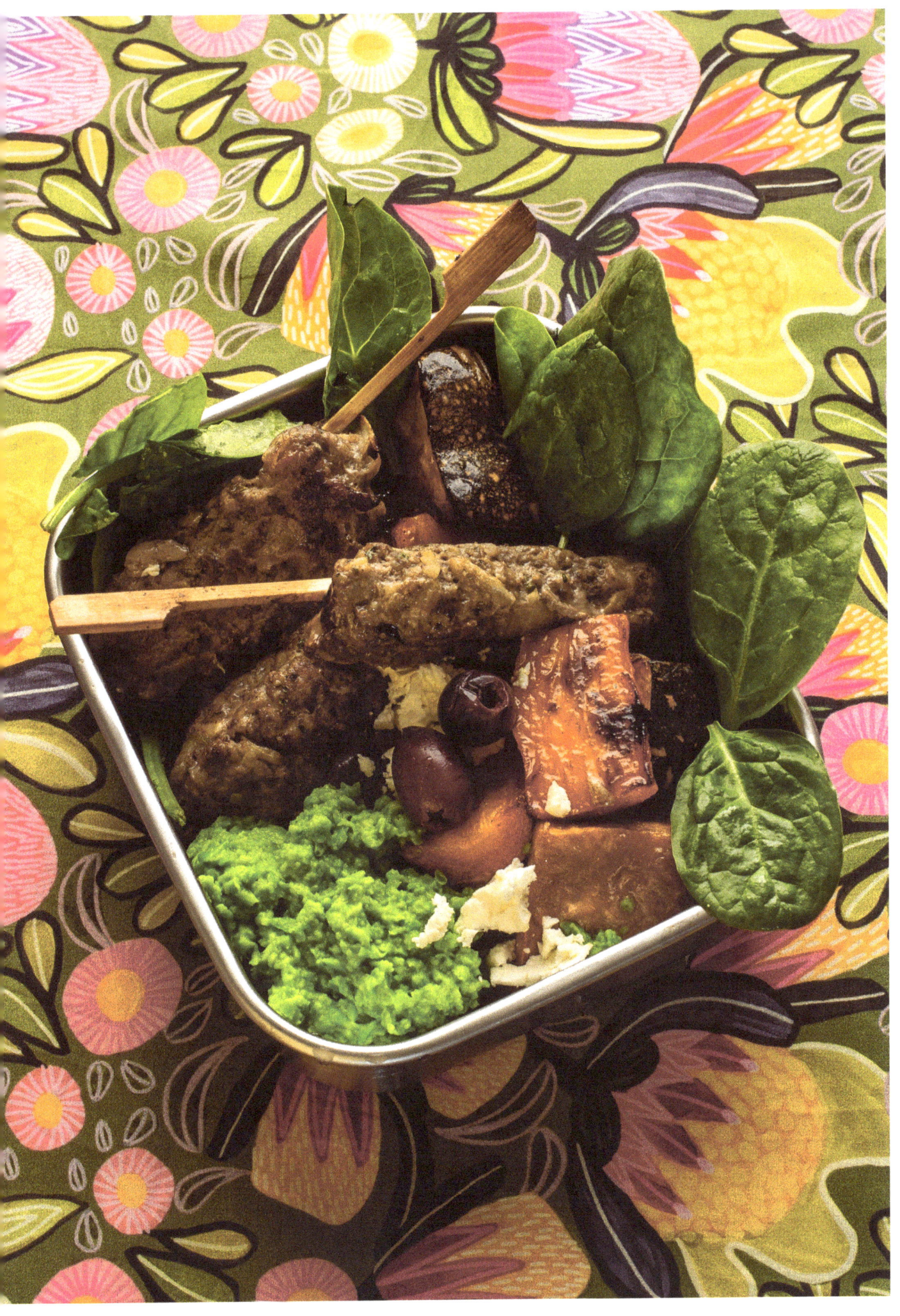

Spicy Lamb Shank

SERVES 4-6

This can be cooked in a 150°C oven in a lidded casserole dish. If using the slow cooker the temperatures and cooking times vary so you'll need to get to know yours. Serve with the quinoa salad (page 126) or mashed spuds and veggies.

3 lamb shanks

2 tablespoon flour
(brown rice flour for GF)

extra virgin olive oil

3 onions

2 carrots

1 teaspoon smoked paprika

½ teaspoon chilli

6 cloves garlic

1 teaspoon pepper

1 teaspoon salt

1 tablespoon parsley

1 tablespoon basil

1 tablespoon oregano

½ teaspoon thyme

400 grams tomatoes

salt and pepper

Roll the shanks in the flour and heat the oil in a heavy based pan and fry the shanks until brown.

Peel and dice the carrot, dice the onion, peel and crush the garlic. Add to the slow cooker with the shanks, tomato, herbs and spices and cook on high for about 4 hours until cooked through and the meat is falling off the bones. Season.

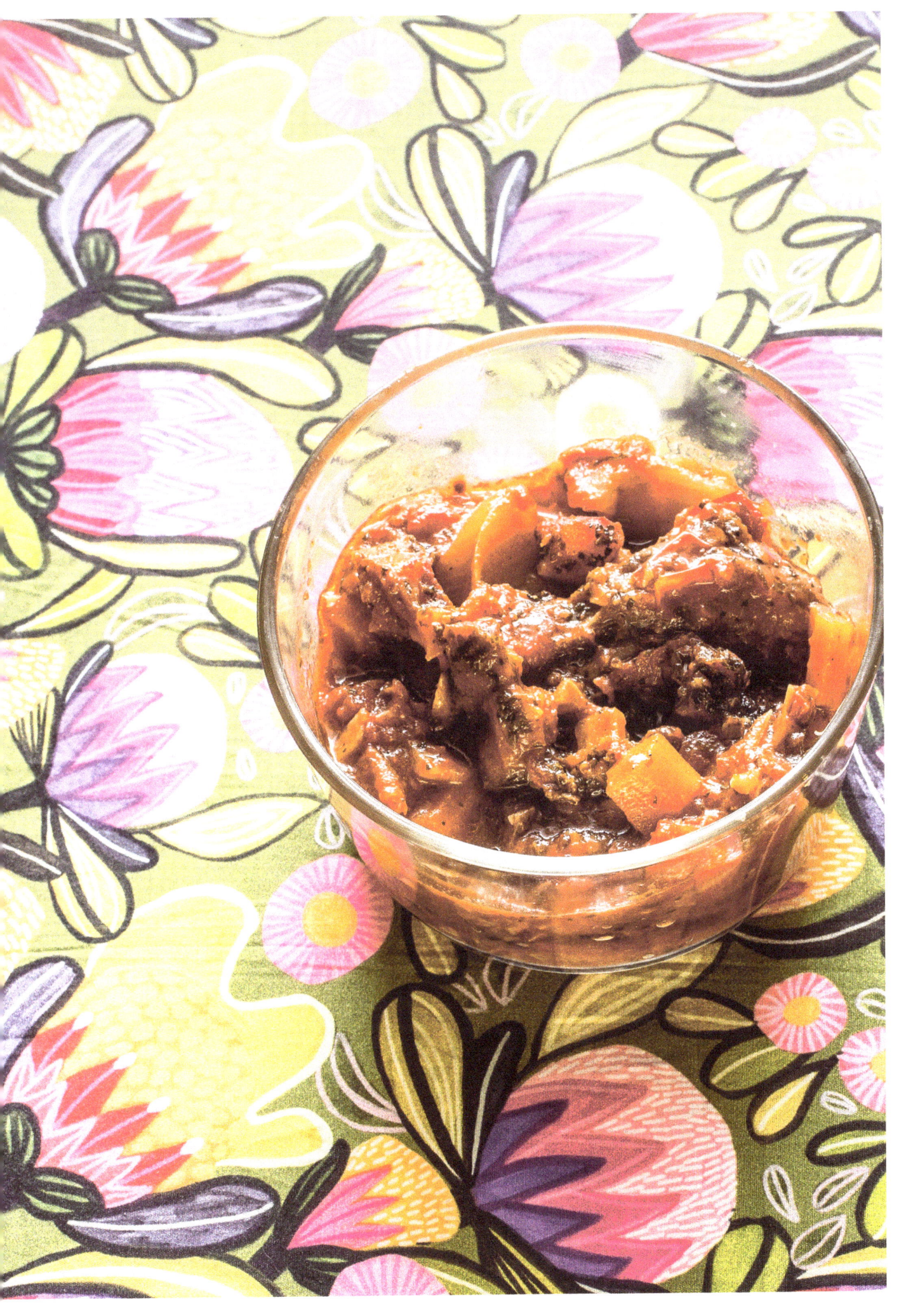

Quinoa Roast Vegetable Salad

SERVES 4-6

Cook quinoa in broth for extra nutrients. I find quinoa simply cooked bland to eat on the side of a casserole in place of rice, but a salad like this is beautiful.

4 large carrots

1 medium sweet potato

1 cup quinoa

3 cups stock

pinch cumin

2 tablespoons extra virgin olive oil

handful fresh mint leaves

handful fresh parsley leaves

100 grams fetta

4 cups spinach leaves

2 tomatoes

1 clove garlic

¼ red onion

Heat the oven to 180°C.

Peel and dice the carrots and sweet potato into a rough 1-2 cm dice and rub in extra virgin olive oil in a roasting dish and roast in the oven for around 20 minutes until cooked. Cool.

To cook the quinoa, simmer in the stock covered for around 15 minutes until cooked. Cool.

Chop tomato, onion and herbs and leaves and crush garlic. Mix all ingredients together with the crumbled fetta and cumin.

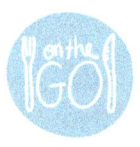

Leave herbs and leaves on top and mix through just before eating.

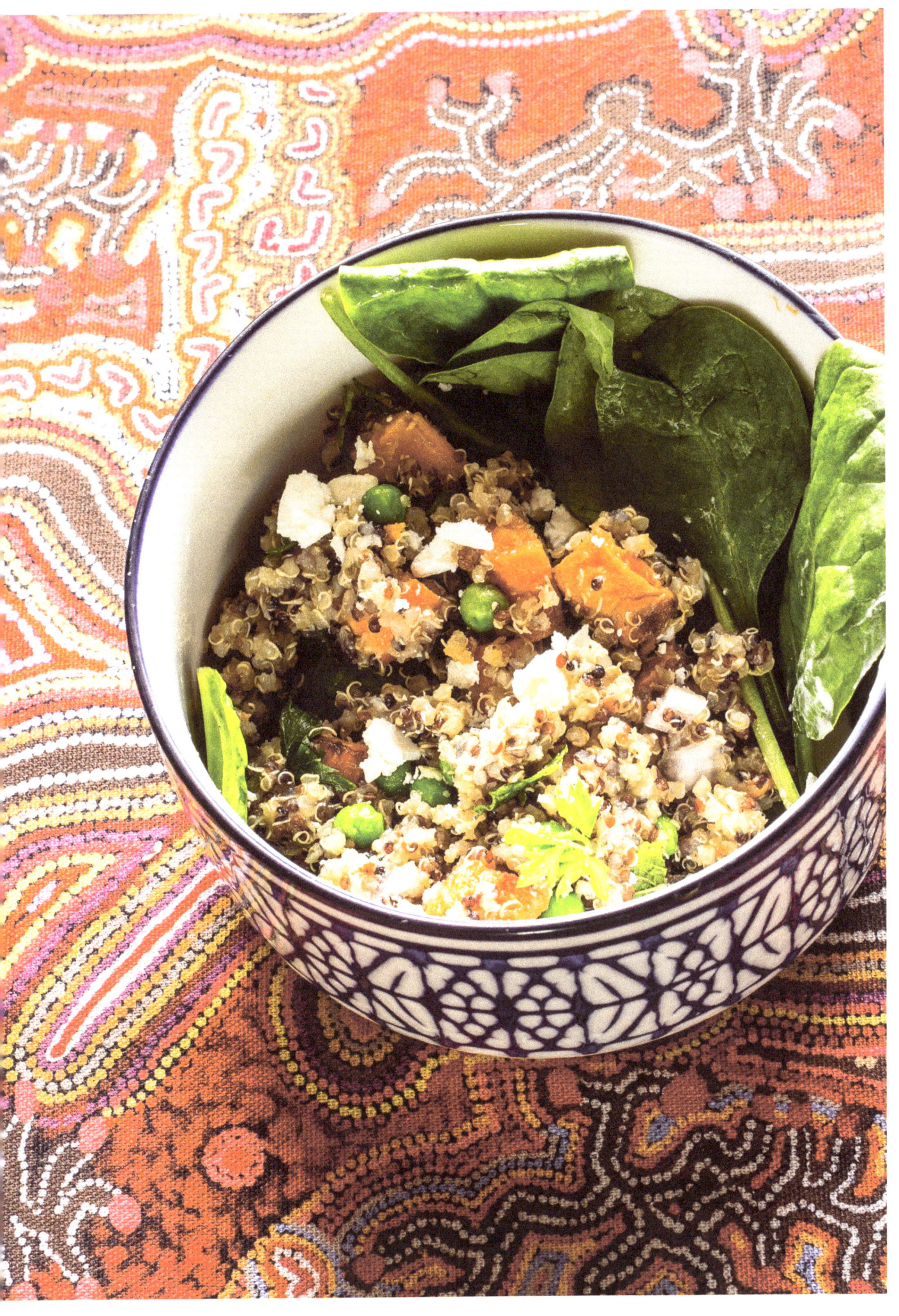

Pesto Mayo Chicken Salad

SERVES 4

PESTO

big bunch basil

50 grams parmesan

100 grams pinenuts

3 cloves garlic

pinch salt

pinch pepper

80ml extra virgin olive oil

SALAD

4 tablespoons pesto

2 tablespoon mayonnaise (see basics page 25)

2 tablespoons sour cream

600 grams chicken thighs

2 cups penne pasta

2 cups spinach

2 cups peas

1 head broccoli

To make the pesto blend all the ingredients in the blender to form a chunky paste. Any left over pesto can be stored in the fridge for a few weeks, make sure the sides of the jar is clean and it has a thin layer of extra virgin olive oil on top and a lid.

Heat the oven to 180°C.

Pop the thighs in a baking dish, rub with extra virgin olive oil and bake in the oven for about 20 minutes until cooked through. Cook the pasta to the packet directions. Steam the broccoli for about 5 minutes until just cooked, then cool. Mix the pesto, mayo and sour cream together in a large bowl. Add the cut chicken, peas, broccoli and spinach, mix well and serve.

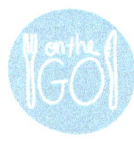

Leave the spinach separately or just sitting in top in the container and mix through just before eating.

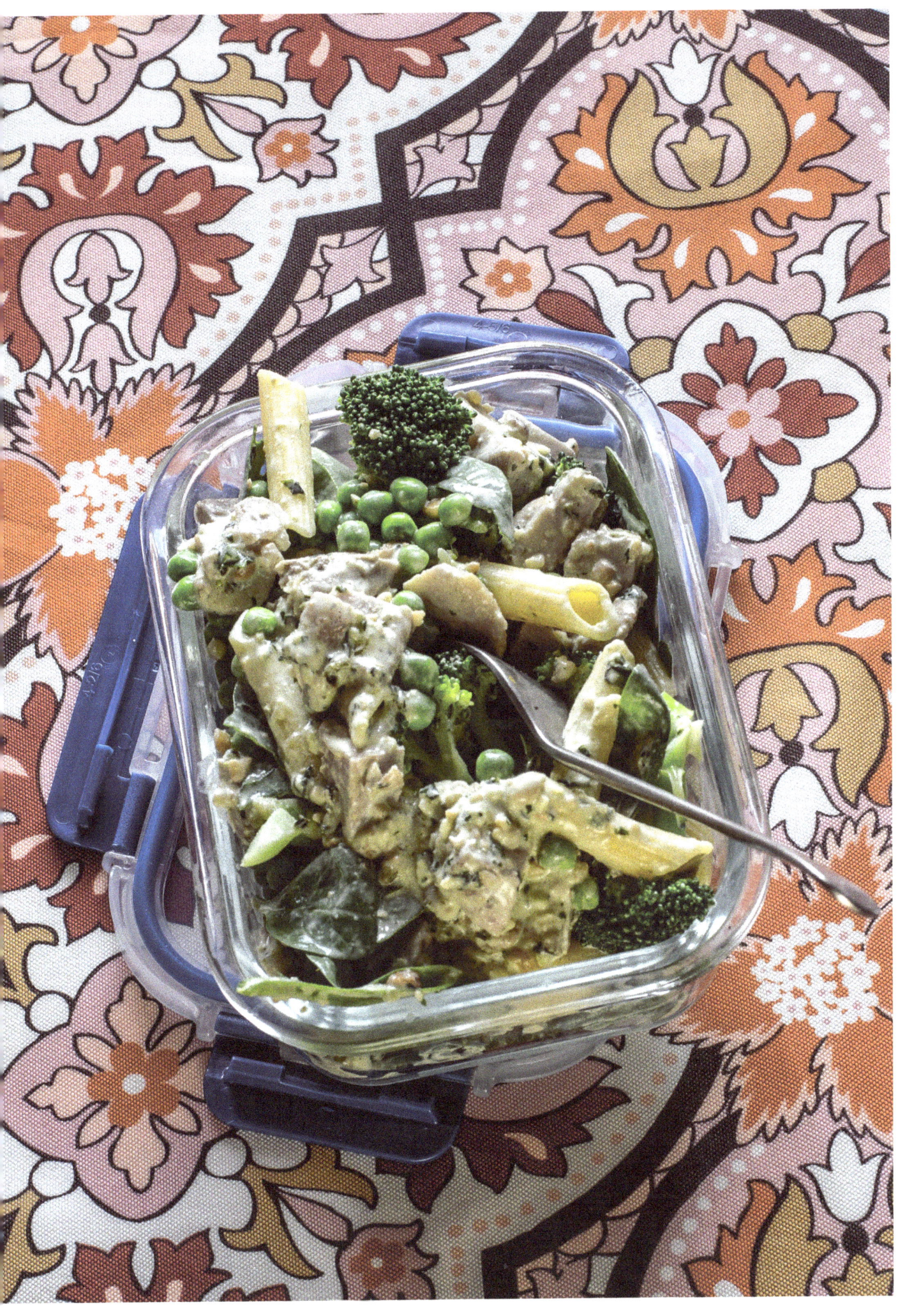

Apple After School Muffins

MAKES ABOUT 18 SMALLS ABOUT 2 TABLESPOONS OF MIX MUFFINS

These dense muffins are a different texture for children, but with a dollop of sweetened cream cheese these will be considered a "treat". Perfect for a nutrient dense quick snack on the school to activities run!

1 cup cooked kidney beans

3 apples

¾ cup chickpea flour

¾ cup cacao

2 tablespoons honey

½ teaspoon cinnamon

1 cup almonds

1 cup dates

3 eggs

2 teaspoons baking powder

½ cup extra virgin olive oil

TOPPING

cream cheese

honey

Heat the oven to 180°C.

Line your muffin trays. I pop all the ingredients in the thermocooker and whip up to a smooth batter in a minute or 2, or you can use your food processor. Pop into the muffin cases and bake for around 20 minutes until cooked through. Cool.

Mix the cream cheese and honey and ice each cupcake.

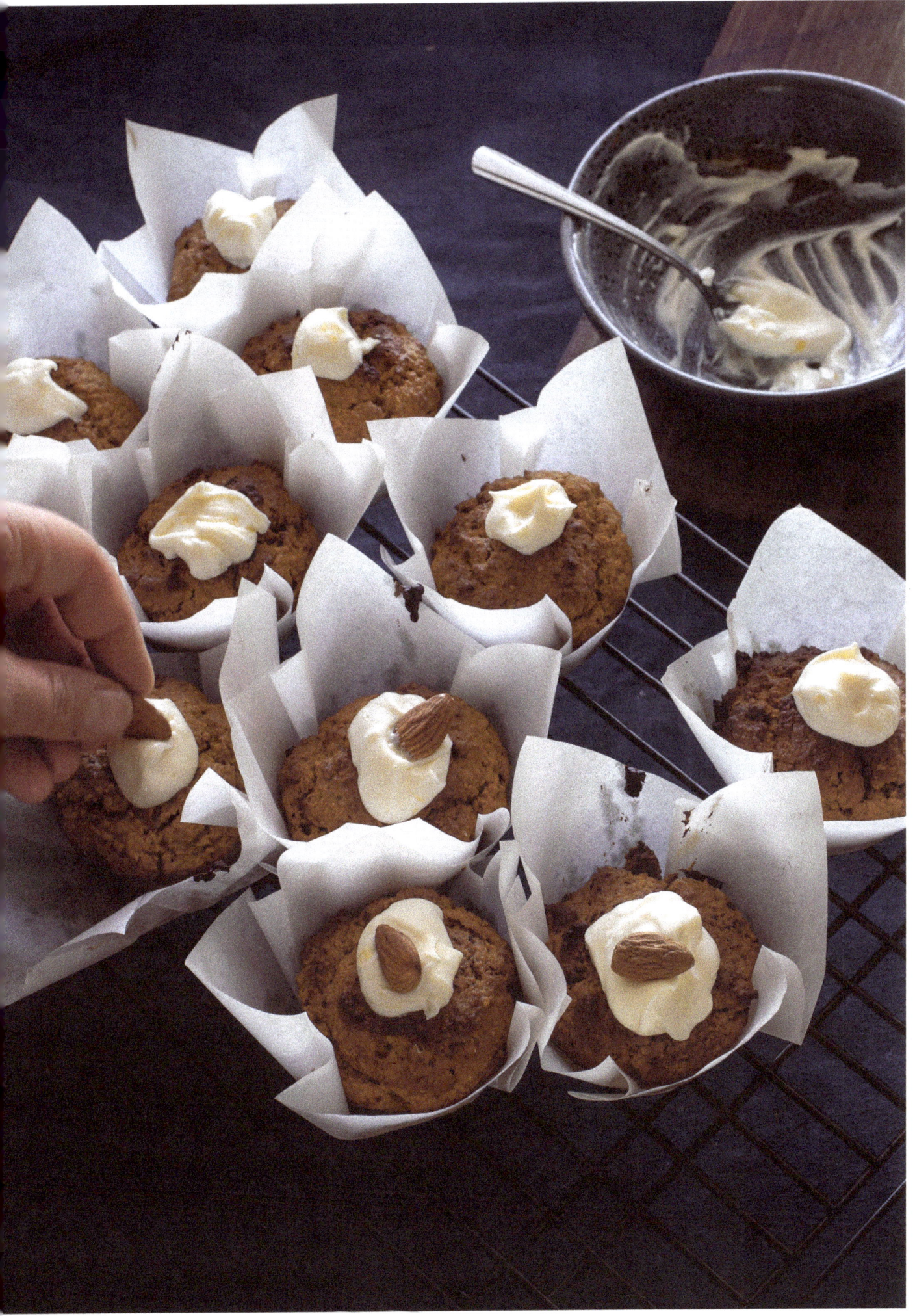

Egg and Bacon Pies

MAKES 12

The pies made with pastry freeze well for a quick lunch to pack, you can use a simple short crust pastry or use a few sheets of good quality frozen puff pastry. Or use the pastry free version or sliced bread version for a quick to prep breakie on a busy morning.

3 sheets of pastry

8 eggs

4 rashers bacon

150ml cream

salt and pepper

150 grams tasty cheese

Heat the oven to 180°C.

Spray muffin trays with oil and cut each sheet of pastry into 4. Line the muffin trays with the pastry. Crack the eggs into a bowl and whisk together with the cream, then season with salt and pepper. Slice the bacon into small pieces and distribute evenly into the pastry cases and pour egg mix over. Top with the grated cheese. Bake for 15- 20 minutes or until golden brown and cooked through.

For a pastry free version simply wrap bacon around the inside of the muffin tin to line, and crack an egg in. You could add tomato, cheese, mushrooms, spinach, olives and more.

Or replace the pastry with a slice of bread that has been rolled out flat and spread with butter to line the muffin tray, crack in an egg and shredded bacon plus cheese, tomatoes, mushrooms and spinach.

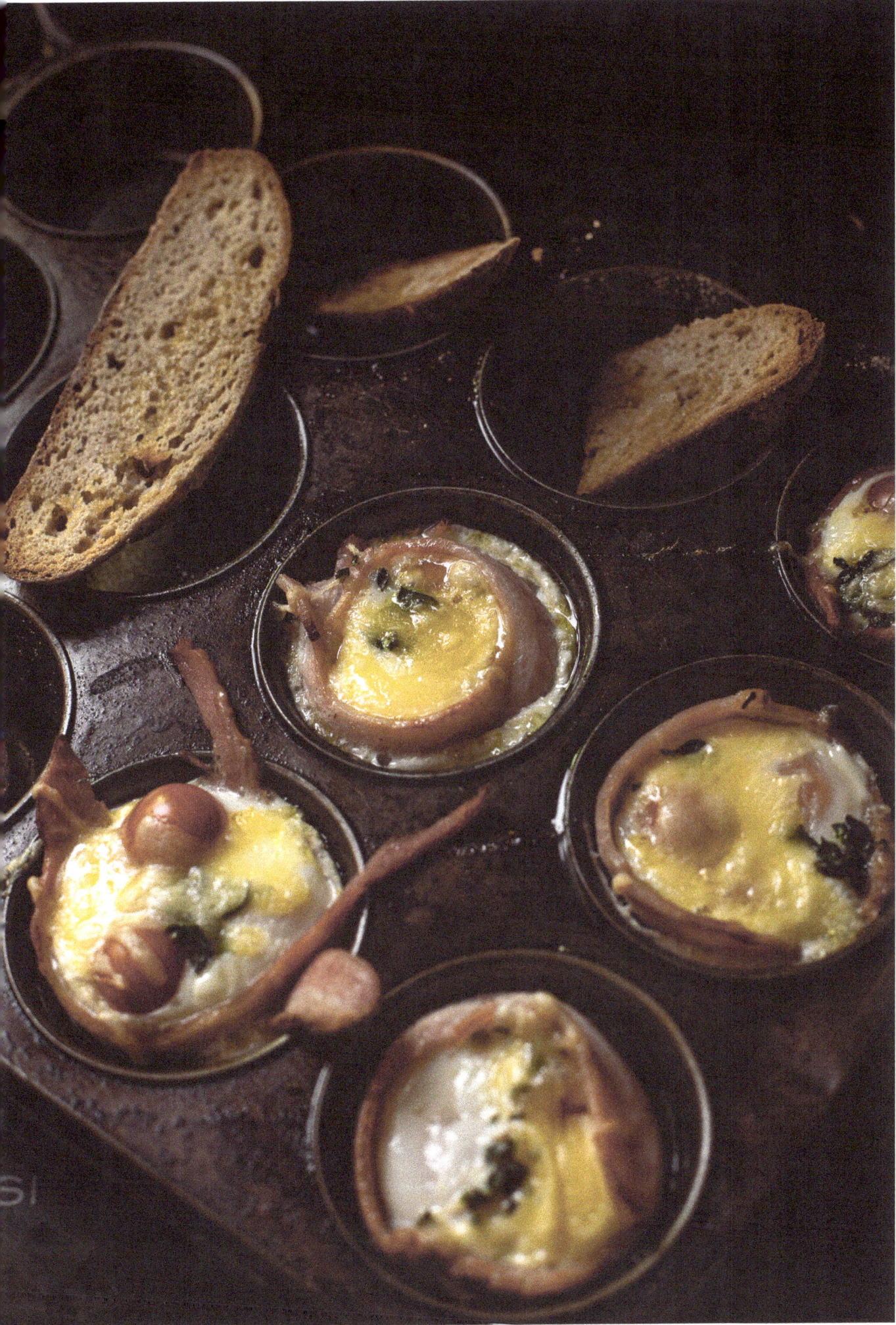

Noodle Salad

SERVES 4-6

This would have to be one of my kids favourite salads, I have left this recipe simple but other veggies you have on hand can be added like capsicum, broccoli or celery. It can be served with chicken, fish and other meats.

2 spring onions

2 medium carrots

2 cup green cabbage

2 cup red cabbage

DRESSING

1 tablespoon soy sauce

1 tablespoon balsamic vinegar

2 tablespoon extra virgin olive oil

2 cloves garlic

1 tablespoon honey

TO SERVE

crunchy or cooked noodles

Grate carrot and finely slice onion and cabbage. Mix all the dressing ingredients together.

Mix all ingredients together and serve.

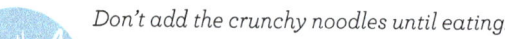

Don't add the crunchy noodles until eating.

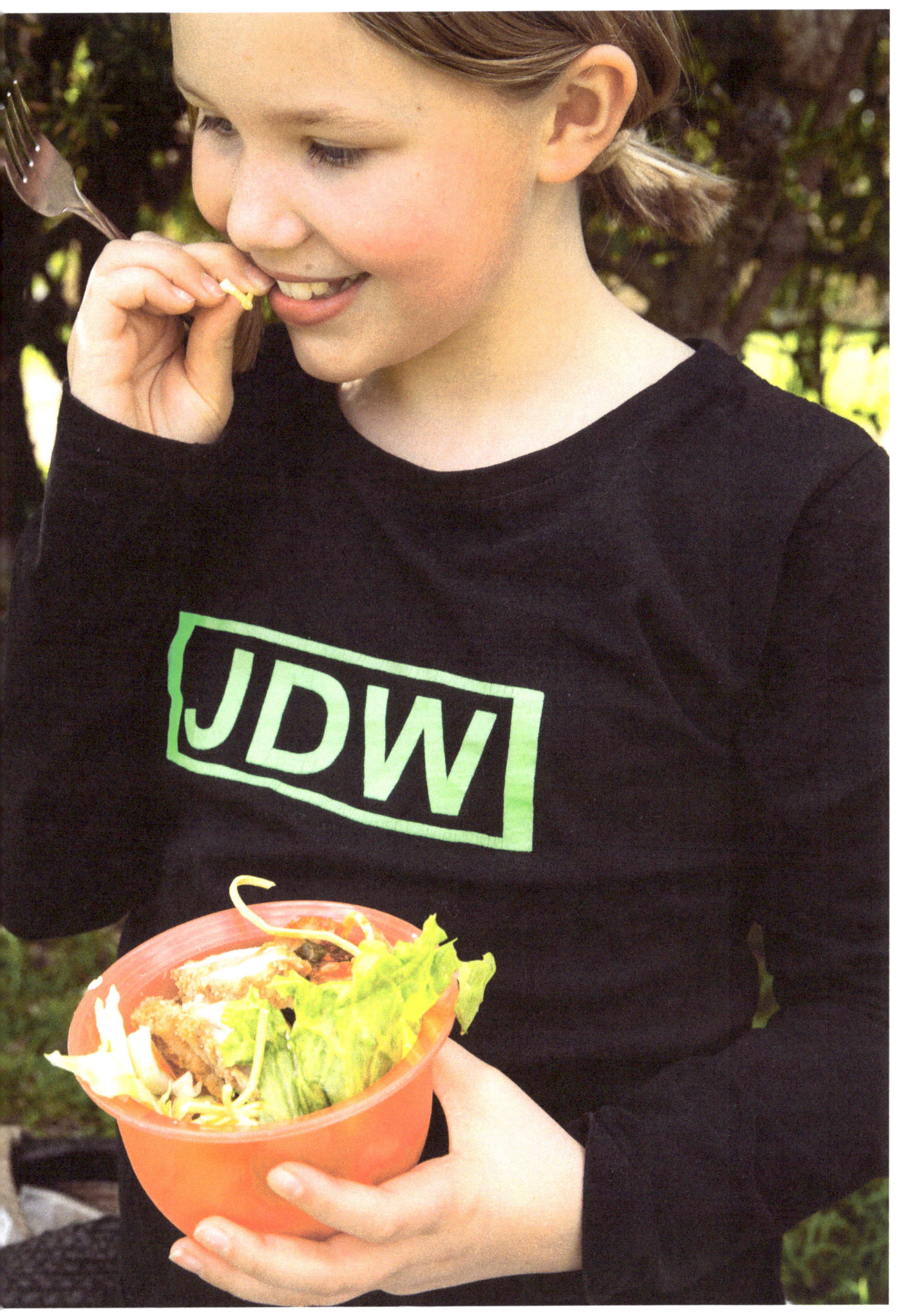

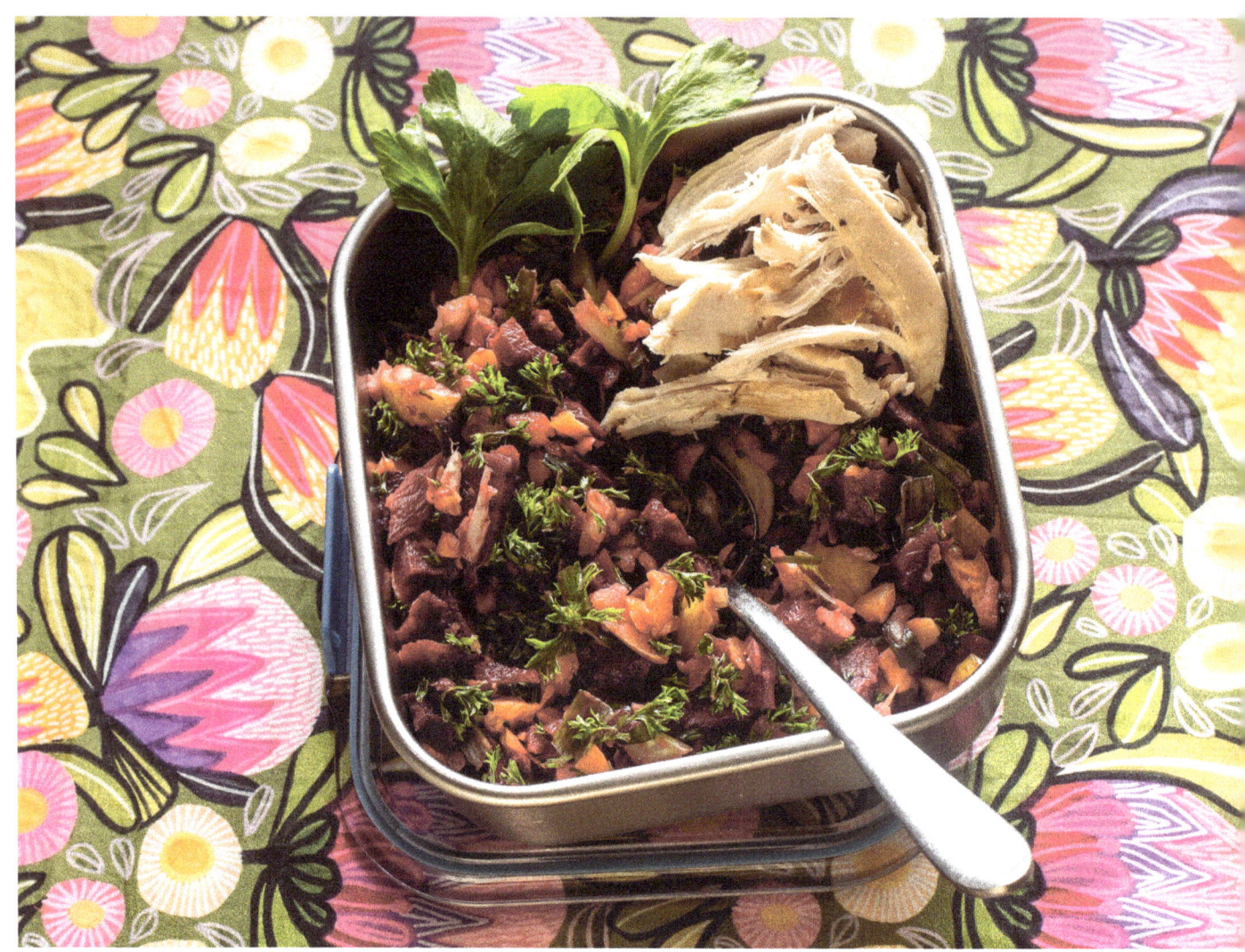

Beetroot Salad

SERVES 4

2 large beetroots

2 carrots

1 apple

2 sticks celery

1 large clove garlic

½ bunch parsley

3 spring onions

extra virgin olive oil

Peel and chop all ingredients and pop into the thermocooker bowl and grate on a low speed SLOWLY so it remains as chunky as you like. Alternatively, you could use another food processor of choice or grate and chop the ingredients by hand.

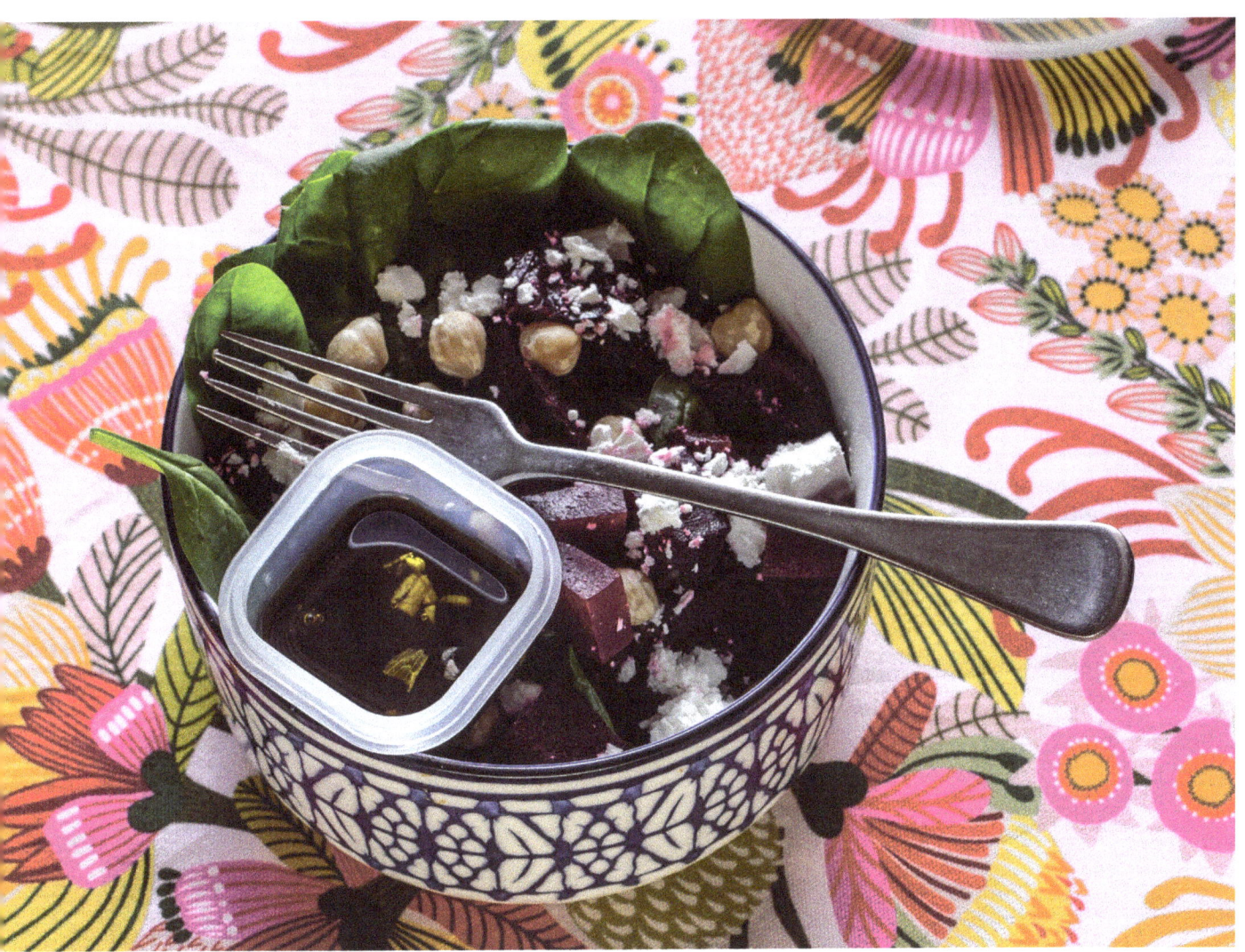

Roast Beetroot and Fetta Salad

SERVES 4

This is super simple and delicious salad to whip up when you have pre-cooked the beetroots.

4 large beetroots

100 grams fetta

100 grams hazelnuts

pepper

4 tablespoons extra virgin olive oil

2 tablespoons balsamic

2 cloves garlic

4 cups spinach

Heat the oven to 180°C.

Rub the beetroots in a little oil and roast in the oven for about 25 minutes until cooked through - there should be little resistance when stabbed with a fork. Cool, peel and dice into 1cm cubes. Mix with the crumbled fetta, nuts and spinach and dress with the crushed garlic, balsamic and oil that has been whisked together well.

Green Chicken Curry

SERVES 4-6

Make this paste, split it into 3 batches and freeze the extra 2 serves for other meals. When I was making it for a restaurant, I would use shrimp paste instead of the fish sauce. As I don't really want a packet of shrimp paste hanging around in the fridge all year at home, I use a dash of fish sauce from the bottle that I use regularly in cooking. I'll sometimes use ground spices at home rather than roasting the seeds and grinding to save time. I have added in an option here to replace the chicken with duck, a vegetable or fish version is nice too!

PASTE (FOR AT LEAST 3 MEALS)

4 cloves garlic

1 tablespoon ginger root

2 sticks lemon grass

1 bunch coriander

½ bunch basil

½ teaspoon ground turmeric

1 teaspoon ground white pepper

2 large green chillies

4 kaffir lime leaves

1 tablespoon fish sauce

1 red onion

½ teaspoon ground cumin

¼ teaspoon ground coriander

extra chilli (optional)

CURRY

600-800 grams chicken thigh or breast or one roast duck

1 onion

500ml vegetable or chicken stock

400ml coconut milk

300 grams cooked noodles

4 cups vegetables such as carrot, capsicum, bok choy, greens, peas, corn, mushrooms, broccoli cauliflower

To make the paste blend all the paste ingredients together.

To cook the curry, slice the onion and cut the chicken into about 1.5cm pieces. Heat a wok over a medium heat until hot, add a dash of oil, add the onion and chicken and sauté for a few minutes until the onion is soft and the chicken is brown. Add hard finely sliced vegetables (carrot, broccoli etc. that take a little longer to cook) and the stock, then simmer until chicken and vegetables are almost cooked (4-6 minutes). Add coconut cream and the soft vegetables (spinach leaves, bok choy leaves that really just need to heat) and noodles and serve when it is all cooked and hot.

*If you want to replace the chicken with roast duck, lay at the bottom on a slow cooker with some chopped up onion, celery and carrot (if you save your peelings from these in a bag in the freezer like I do grab a few handfuls of this instead) put the duck on top breast side up, season well with salt and pepper and leave to cook on high for 4-6 hours until cooked through.

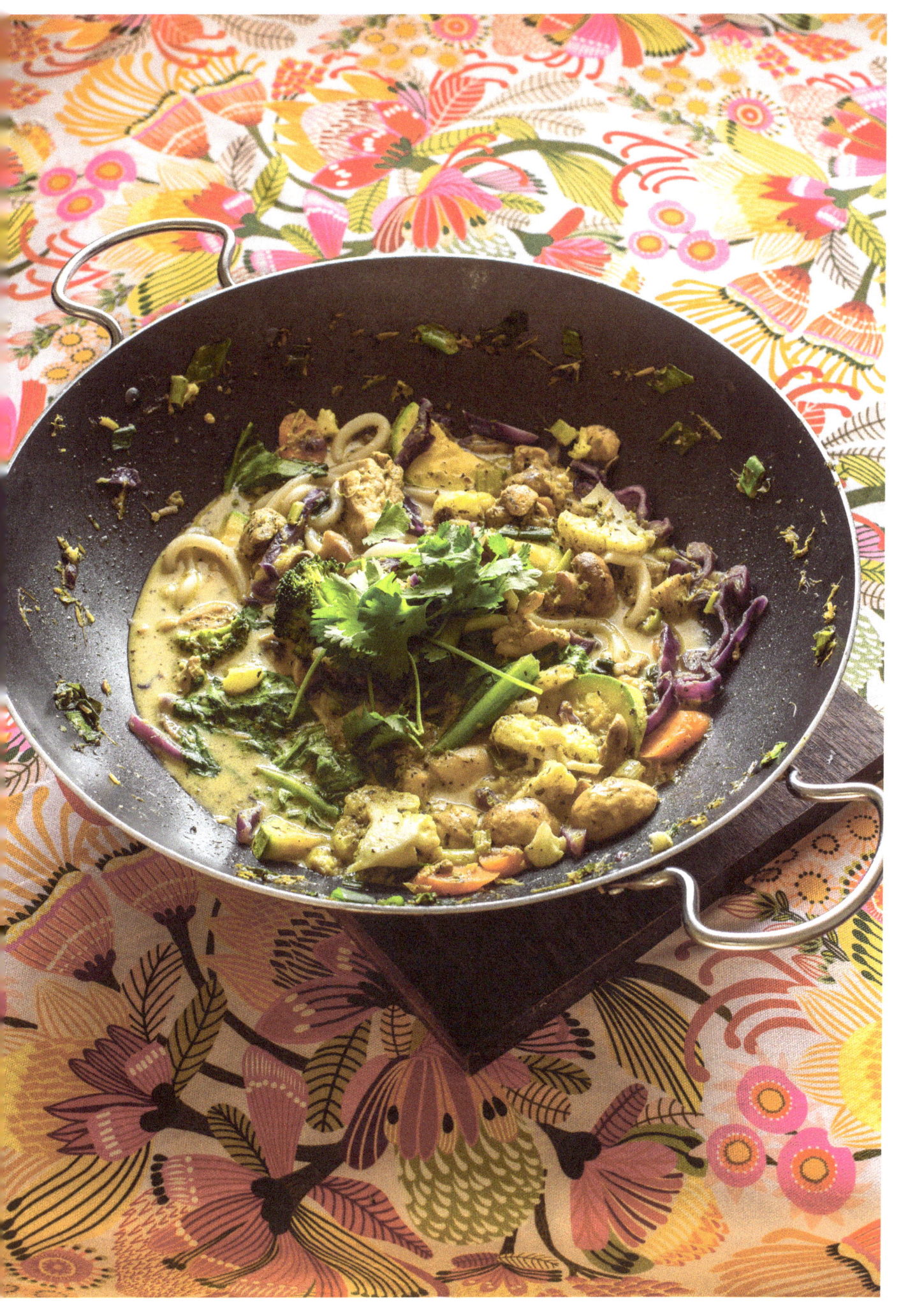

Mexican Meatballs

SERVES 4-6

500 grams beef mince

1 onion

2 cloves garlic

1 tablespoon oregano

1 tablespoon smoked paprika

1 tablespoon cumin

1 teaspoon cinnamon

½ teaspoon sea salt

½ teaspoon cracked black pepper

fresh or dried chillies to taste

1 egg

1 cup fresh bread crumbs

Dice onion and crush garlic and mix all ingredients together well. Roll into balls and pan fry in a large heavy based pan over a medium heat until cooked through. Serve hot or cold with a dipping salsa or with corn chips, salsa and guacamole.

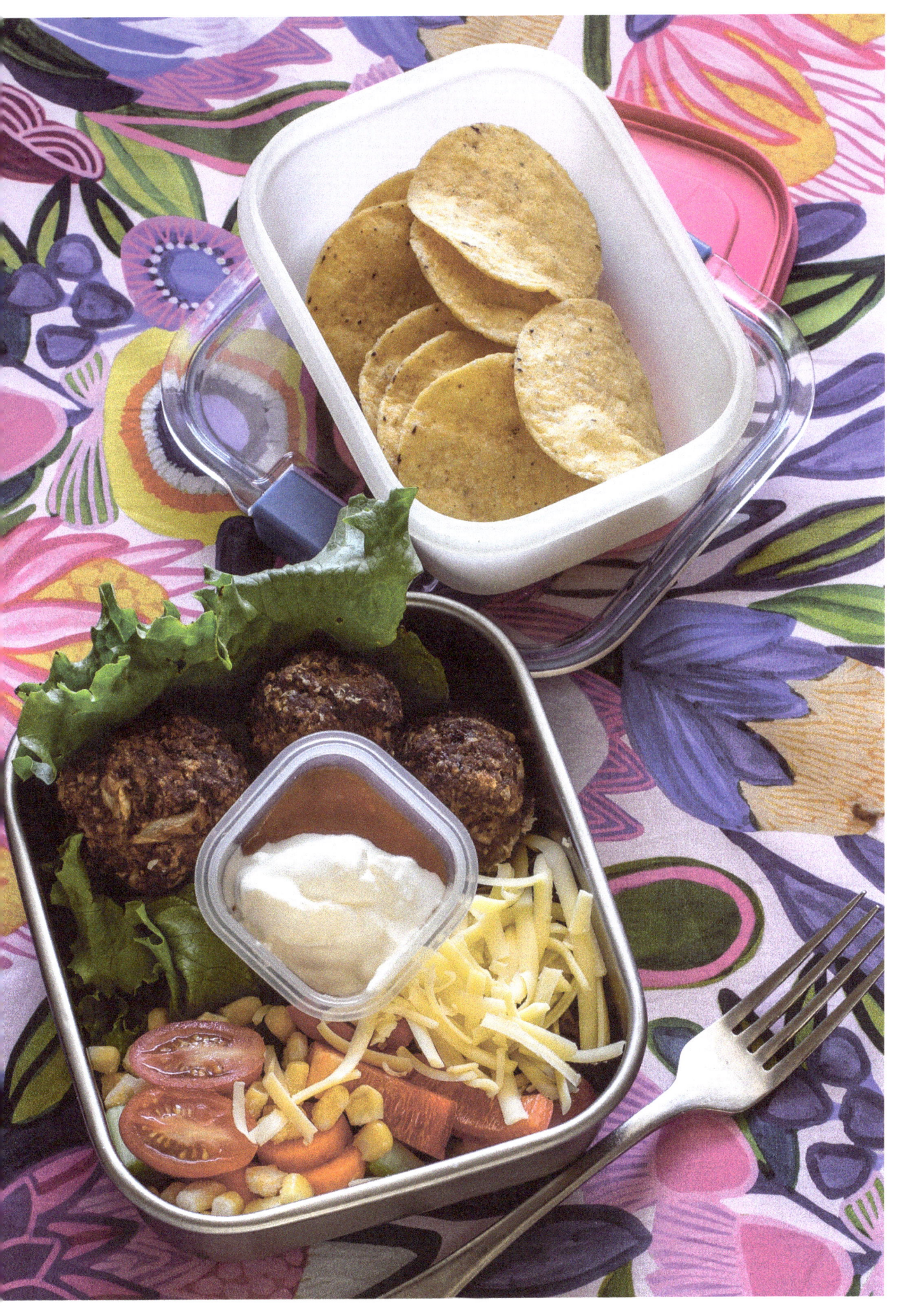

Sichuan Pepper Pork Salad

SERVES 4

This is delicious with the pork steak cooked and served hot, but a dish that is equally delicious cold, so a good one for a hearty and filling cold packed dinner. You could also try chicken, salmon, or a thin egg omelette as the protein in this or add some nuts and keep it vego!

600 grams thin sliced pork scotch or loin or fillet

2 tablespoons soy sauce

4 cloves garlic

2cm chunk ginger

2 tablespoons sesame oil

½ teaspoon sichuan pepper

½ teaspoon Chinese 5 spice

2 cups rice noodles

2 carrots

1 cucumber

4 handfuls spinach

4 spring onions

fresh chilli to your preference

DRESSING

1 tablespoon soy sauce

1 tablespoon balsamic vinegar

1 tablespoon sesame oil

1 tablespoon extra virgin olive oil

1 clove garlic

Crush the garlic and ginger and mix with the soy, crushed peppers, five spice and sesame and leave to marinate at least overnight.

Soak the rice noodles in boiling water, cool under cold water and drain. Peel and slice all salad ingredients. Mix the dressing ingredients together well. Dress the salad close to eating.

Pan fry the pork in a medium high heat in a pan until cooked through. Rest and serve or cool to pack.

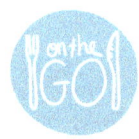

Cook and serve cold but leave the dressing on the side to dress just before eating.

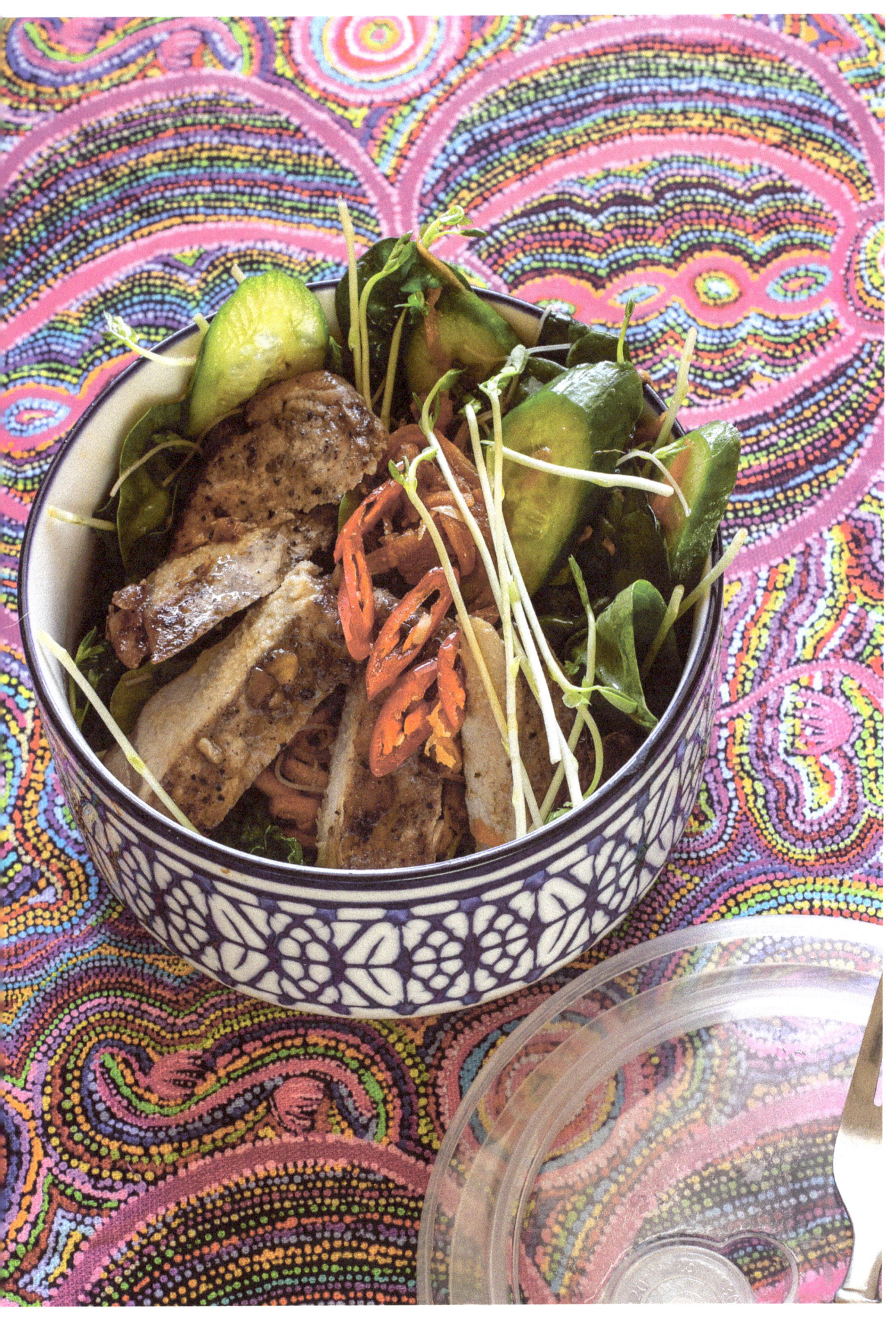

Pickled Octopus, Roast Pumpkin, Fetta

SERVES 4 WITH LEFTOVER PICKLED OCTOPUS

Octopus makes a brilliant protein for a cold packed lunch - you'll find plenty of ideas in all my books!. Low fat, high protein and full of good nutrients we need to thrive. Add extra roast pumpkin to the Sunday roast to make this a quick meal to whip up during the week.

PICKLED OCTOPUS

1 onion

1 teaspoon garlic

1 large chilli

1 teaspoon oregano

1 lemon diced

1 kilogram octopus, cleaned and cut into 10cm pieces

½ teaspoon salt

½ teaspoon pepper

1 litre extra virgin olive oil (approximately)

400 grams pumpkin

4 cups spinach or lettuce

100 grams fetta

DRESSING

½ cup basil

3 cloves garlic

2 sprigs oregano

juice of 1 lemon

2 tablespoons extra virgin olive oil

To pickle the octopus, roughly chop the onion, garlic, chilli and oregano. Using a heavy-based saucepan, heat 1 teaspoon of the extra virgin olive oil over medium heat and sauté the onion, garlic, chilli and oregano for a few minutes, or until the onions have softened. Add the octopus, and stir and fry until all of the surfaces are sealed. Add the lemon, season with salt and pepper, reduce the heat and cook gently for 5 minutes or until a lot of the liquid has come out of the octopus.

Top with enough oil to completely cover the octopus. Reduce heat to low and cook for 40 minutes, simmering gently. Cut a piece of octopus to test if it is cooked – it should be soft, opaque and cooked through. Remove the saucepan from the heat, cover with a lid and set aside to tenderise and cool for at least 3 hours. Once cooled, place in the refrigerator.

Heat the oven to 180°C.

Roast the pumpkin by peeling and chopping into a rough 2 cm dice. Make the dressing by peeling and crushing the garlic and chopping the herbs mix with the lemon and oil. Mix the cooled pumpkin with the spinach, fetta and octopus dress and serve.

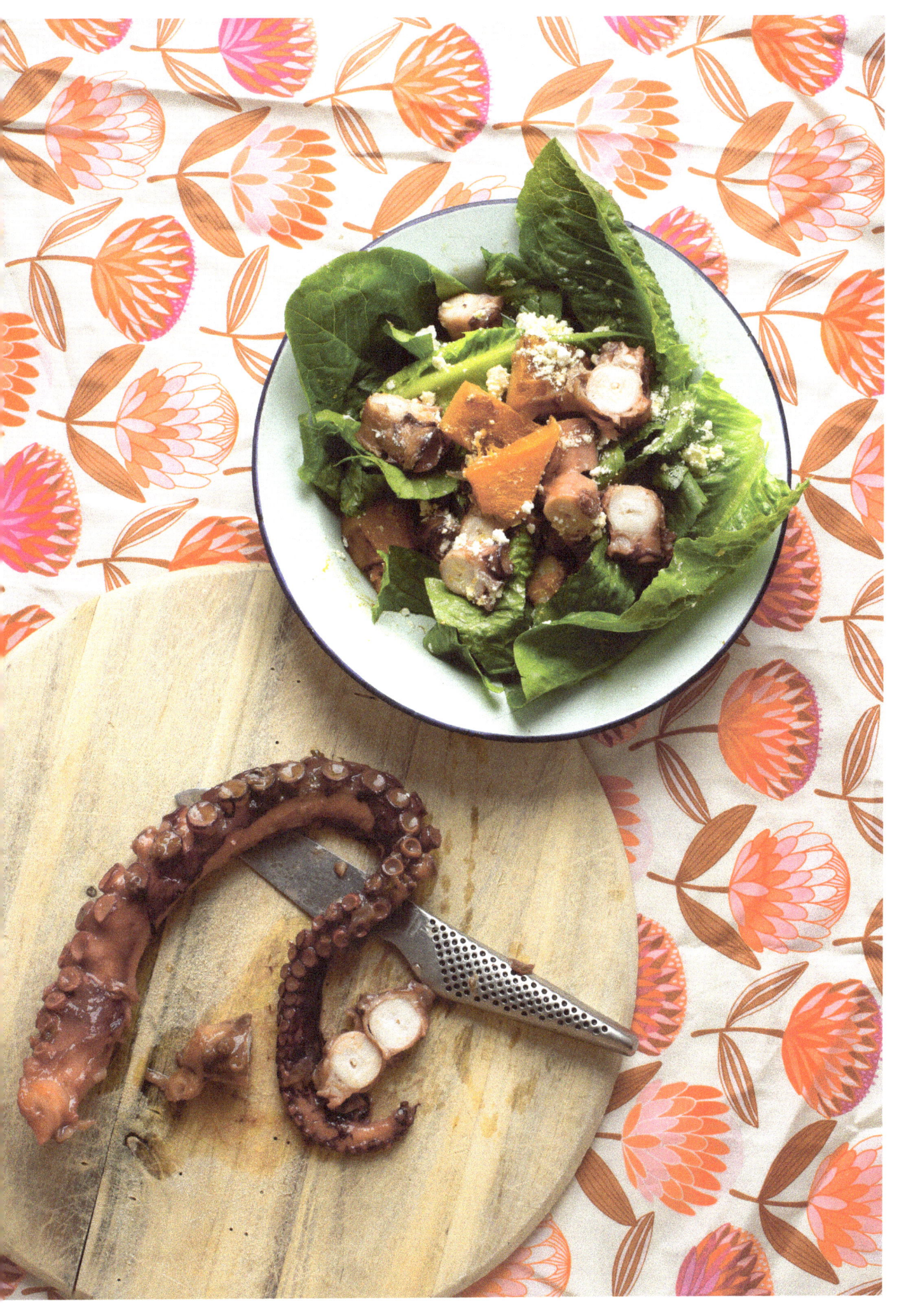

Italian Chicken Meat Balls

SERVES 4

Serve with pesto or tapenade and a simple green salad or in a chilled pasta salad. These meatballs make a handy after school snack for kids heading off to a few hours of sport!

500 grams chicken mince

3 cloves garlic

1 onion

1 tablespoon basil

1 tablespoon oregano

1 teaspoon fennel

½ cup sundried tomato

2 tablespoons parmesan

pinch pepper

salt

1 egg

1 cup breadcrumbs

extra virgin olive oil

Heat the oven to 180°C.

Finely dice the onion and crush the garlic and pop them in a large bowl. Add the chopped basil, oregano, sundried tomato, fennel, parmesan, breadcrumbs, pepper, salt and egg and mix well. Roll into 2cm balls. Heat the oil in a large heavy based oven proof pan and fry the meat balls making sure there is a bit of space between them in the pan.

When they have some nice brown colour pop the pan in the oven to finish cooking them through for about 15 minutes or until they are cooked through. Serve hot or cold.

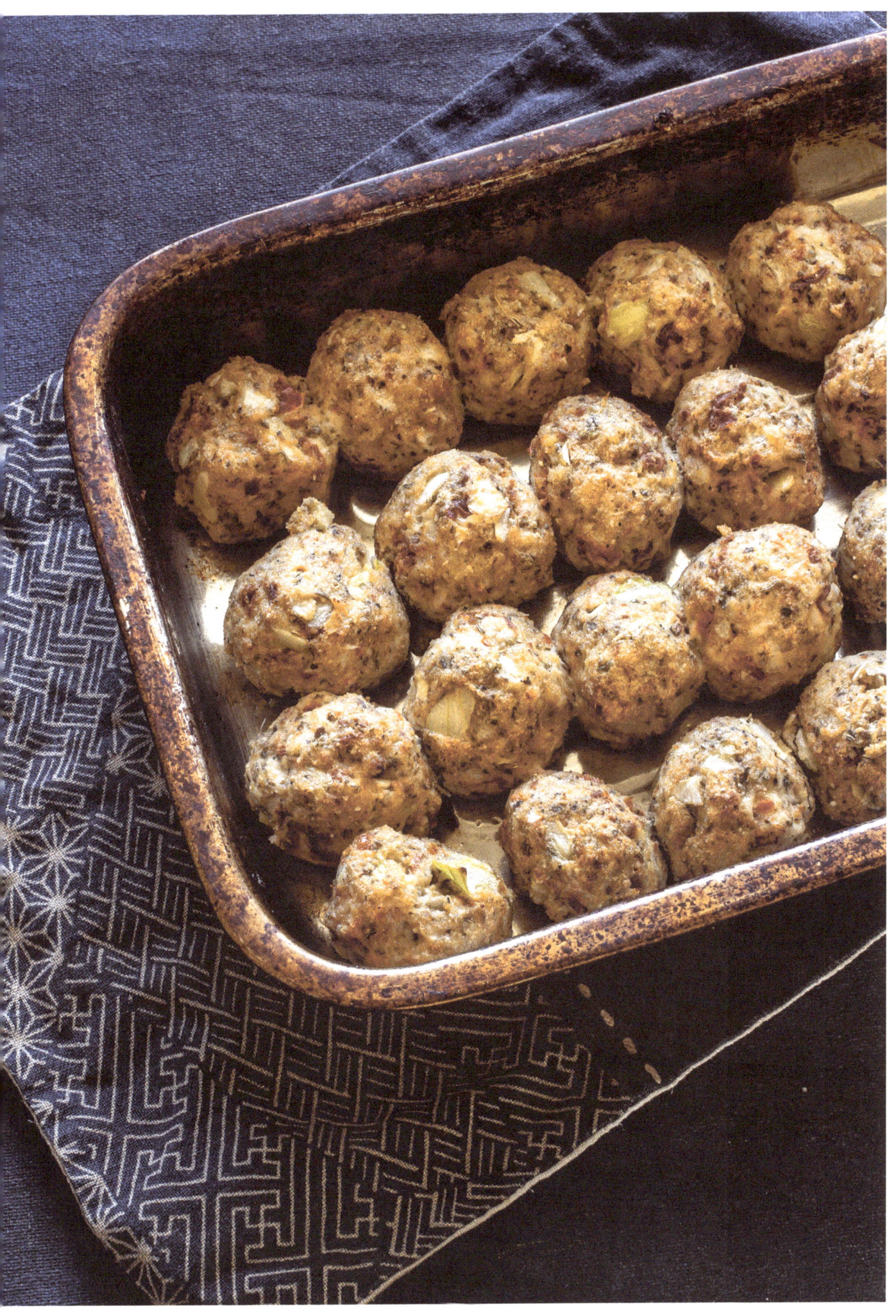

Spicy Breakfast Scones

MAKES 12

There are loads of different ideas for flavours you can use for this tasty grab and go breakfast choice idea. Sundried tomato, olives, different herbs, different cured meats like chorizo sausage, cheeses and more! They are nice served on the side of a soup for lunch too.

3 cups self-raising flour

1 teaspoon salt

50 grams butter

2 tablespoons chives

1 tablespoon thyme

2 tablespoons parsley

100 grams fetta

200 grams bacon

80 grams pickled jalapenos

smoked paprika

pinch pepper

1 ½ cups milk

extra butter to serve (optional)

Heat the oven to 180°C.

Line a baking tray with baking paper. Measure the flour and salt into a large mixing bowl. Measure and add the butter and then using your hands rub the butter into the flour until it is well combined. Add the chives, parsley, thyme, chopped bacon, jalapenos, paprika, fetta and pepper and the milk, and mix well until the dough is light but firm. Flatten the dough to about 2cm in thickness and then cut into rounds with a scone cutter.

Grease a baking tray and then place the scones onto the tray, allowing some space between each scone (they will expand during baking). Brush the tops with a little milk and bake them for about 20 minutes or until golden brown and cooked through.

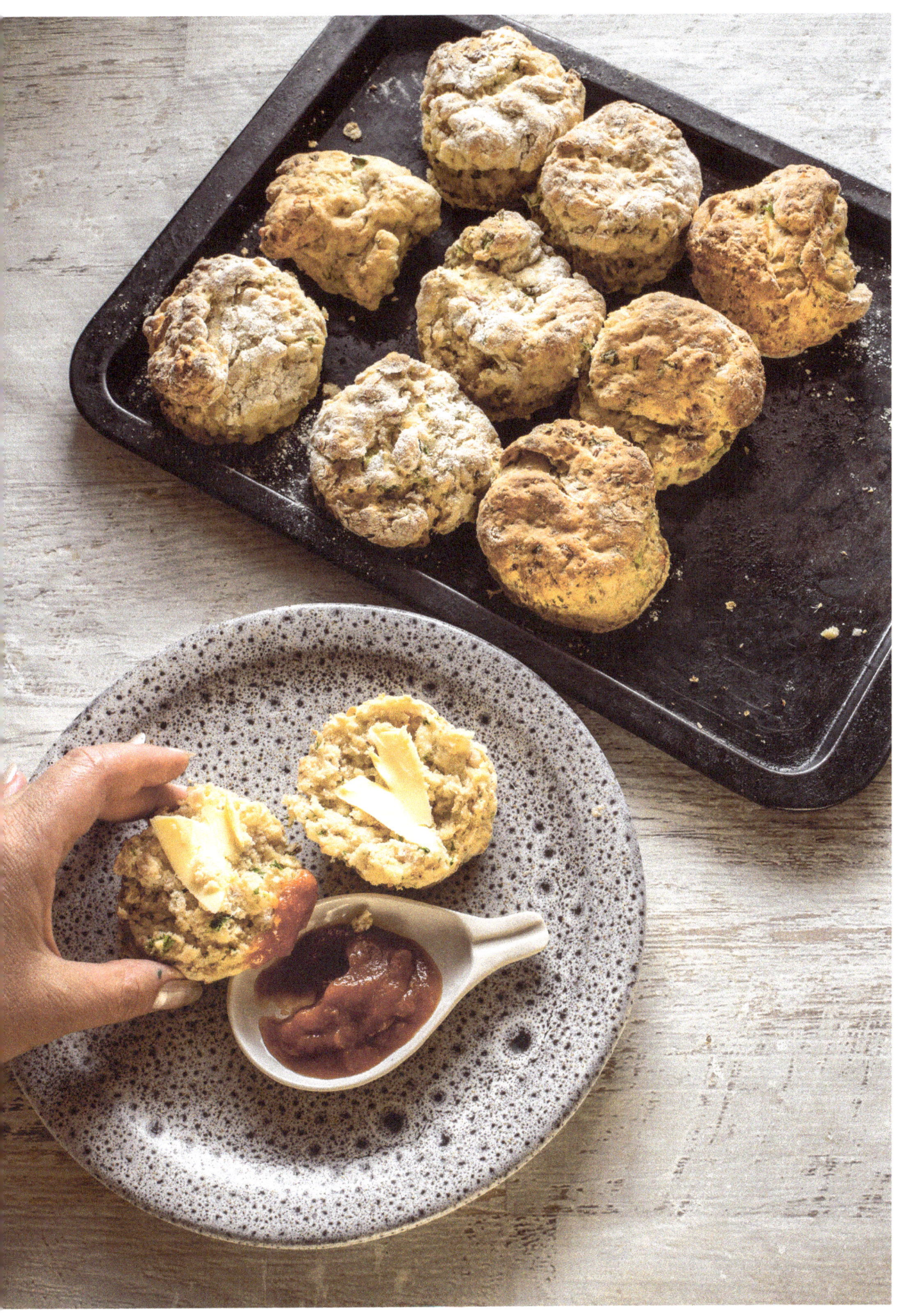

Roast Pumpkin Spinach and Fetta Frittata

SERVES 6-8

The ideas for what to put in the frittata are endless. Bacon and cheese, beetroot and goats cheese, salmon, leftover roast meats. Any leftover roast or steamed veggies from a meal can be popped in a baking dish into the fridge ready to crack a few eggs to make this for a hot breakie or packed lunch with a delicious chutney!

12 eggs
3 cups pumpkin
100ml cream
1 small onion
2 cloves garlic
2 bunches spinach
2 tablespoons basil
50 grams fetta
50 grams parmesan
salt and pepper

Heat the oven to 180°C.

Peel the pumpkin and cut into a rough 1 cm dice, drizzle with extra virgin olive oil and place in a baking dish and bake for 30 minutes or until cooked through. Crack the eggs into a large bowl. Crush the garlic, finely dice the onion finely chop the spinach and basil and add to the egg and mix all ingredients together well with the grated and crumbled cheeses. Pour into a pie dish or baking tray and bake for 20-30 minutes. Serve with chutney and salad.

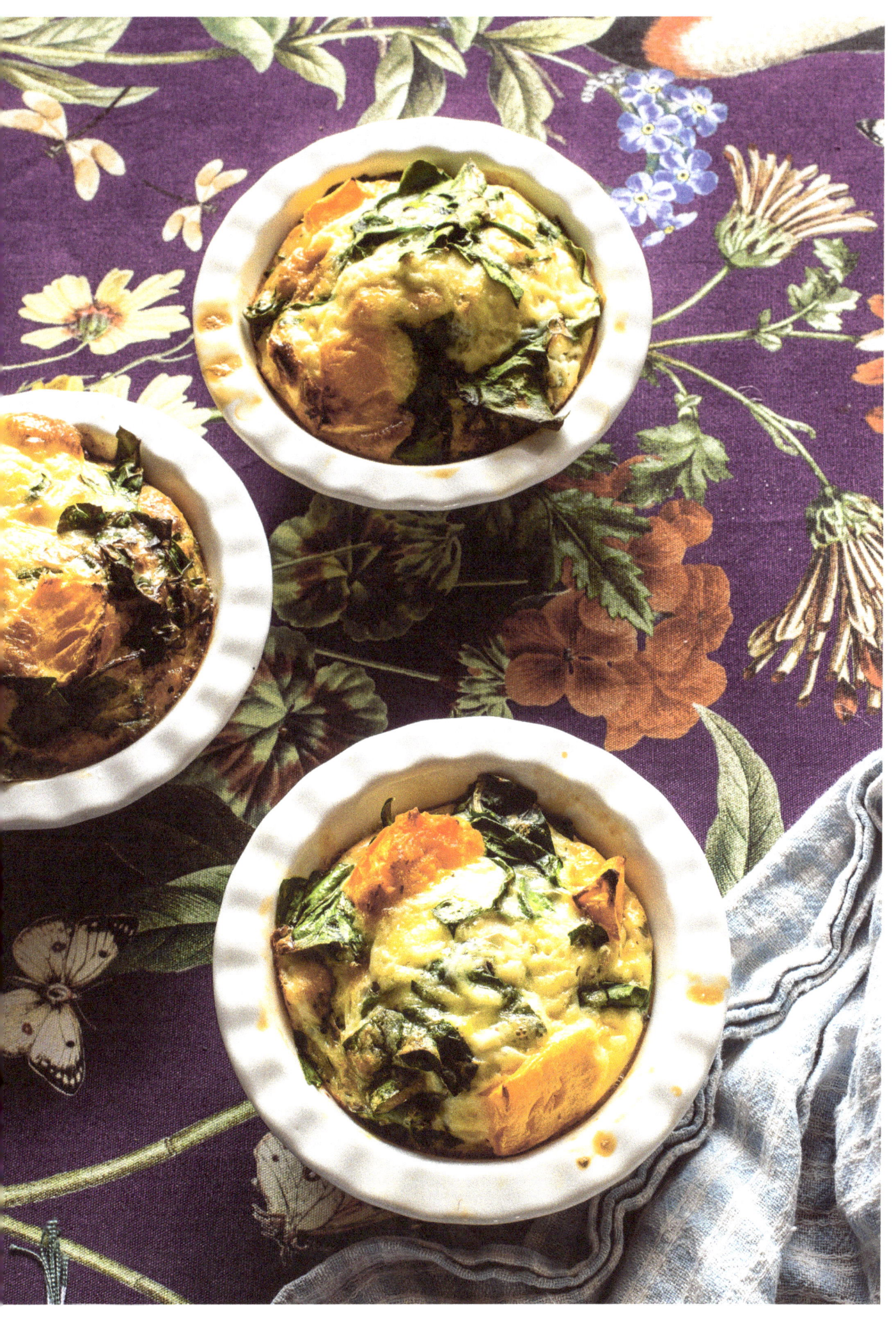

Chicken, Brown Rice and Corn Soup

MAKES 2-3 FAMILY MEALS

I collect the trimmings from my cooking - I was trained during my chef apprenticeship 'old school style', nothing was wasted so there was always an impossible to lift, stock pot or two on the back of the stove to add trimmings to as you chop - but at home I put them in a bag in the freezer. So, when I want to make a stock I grab a few handfuls and add some bay leaves, thyme and peppercorns and any vegetables that may be missing form my trimmings and cover the chicken with water. The stock smells amazing when cooking and it's so nice to have a delicious meal to come home to on a late, cold dark evening after kid's activities. My kids also love this, its full of veggies and they love Italian version with beans and pasta from the same stock. It would be on our weekly meal plan pretty much every week during the school term.

STOCK/BROTH

chicken

500 grams vegetable trimmings of celery, carrot, onion leek

peppercorns

2 bay leaves

3 sprigs thyme

SOUP

3 carrots

2 onions

3 cloves garlic

2 cm piece ginger

2 stalks celery

1 cup cabbage

pinch chilli

1 teaspoon cumin

½ teaspoon garam masala

splash oil

1 cup brown rice

4 cobs corn
(or frozen or tinned kernels corn)

kaffir lime leaf

splash soy and fish sauce

extra vegetables such as spinach, peas, zucchini, broccoli, corn, bok choy, kale, capsicum, mushrooms

salt and pepper

To make the stock: Put the chicken trimmings and herbs and pepper in the slow cooker and cover with water. Simmer in the slow cooker for around 4-6 hours its ready when all the meats falling off the chicken. Strain the chicken and keep the stock and pull all meat from the bones, this meat can be used in salads, wraps or sandwiches or just back into the soup

Peel and mince the garlic and ginger. Peel and dice the carrots, celery, onions and sauté them all in a heavy based pot with the oil, ginger and garlic and the spices and chilli.

Remember to keep all your peelings and trimming to go back into the bag in the freezer for the next to make stock!

Add the rice, corn that has been taken from the cob and blitzed in a food processor, kaffir lime leaf and stock, fish sauce and soy to the pot and gently simmer until the rice is nearly cooked. Now add any extra vegetables that do not require too much cooking.

Easy, super economical and delicious!

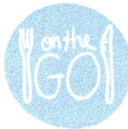 *A thermos full of this delicious soup is amazing on a cold winters day.*

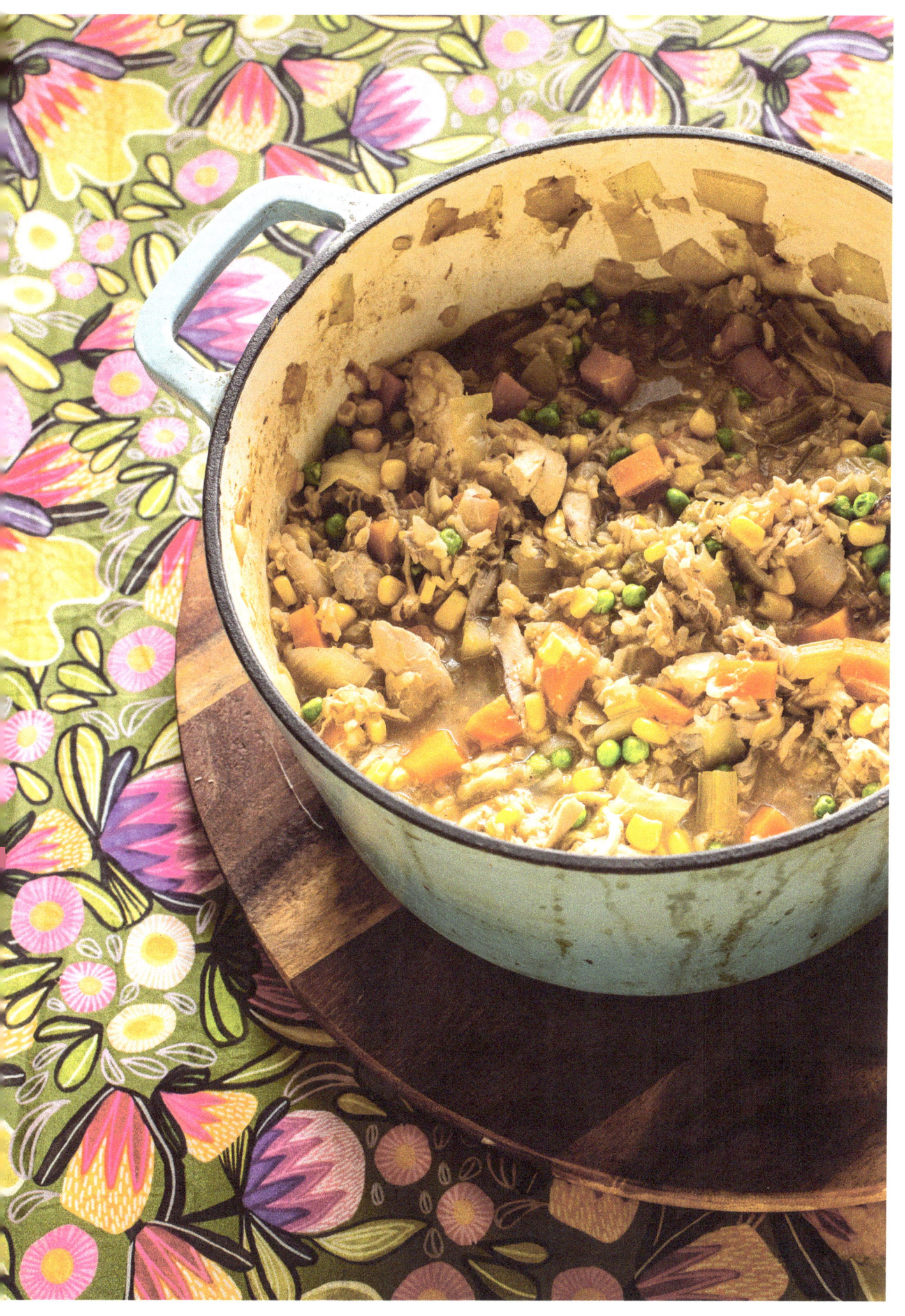

Madras Beef or Lamb Curry

SERVES 6-8

This is one curry that may surprise you at how easy it is to prepare the spice mix for such a tasty meal with so few simple pantry ingredients. Roast and grind your own spices if you have the time and equipment to do so, but I mostly use ground spices at home for ease. The added bonus of a curry is that it will improve in flavour as it sits, so prepare it on the weekend for a busy weeknight meal. For these reasons this curry, with some rice and steamed greens, is on the menu most weeks during winter.

2 brown onions

1 clove garlic

1 tablespoon butter

1 teaspoon turmeric

2 tablespoons ground coriander

1 tablespoon ground cumin

½ teaspoon black pepper

1 teaspoon ground ginger

½ teaspoon chilli flakes

1 tablespoon lemon juice

1 kilo stewing steak or lamb

400 grams crushed tomatoes

1 tablespoon tomato paste

200ml beef stock

Heat the oven to 160°C.

Dice the meat into about a 1.5cm dice. Brown the meat on all sides in batches in a hot pan on the stove top. In a heavy based oven proof sauce pan sauté the diced onion and crushed garlic in the butter for a few minutes until soft add the spices and cook for a few minutes add all the other ingredients and braise covered in the oven for 1-2 hrs until tender.

Or put all ingredients in the slow cooker on high for 4-6 hours.

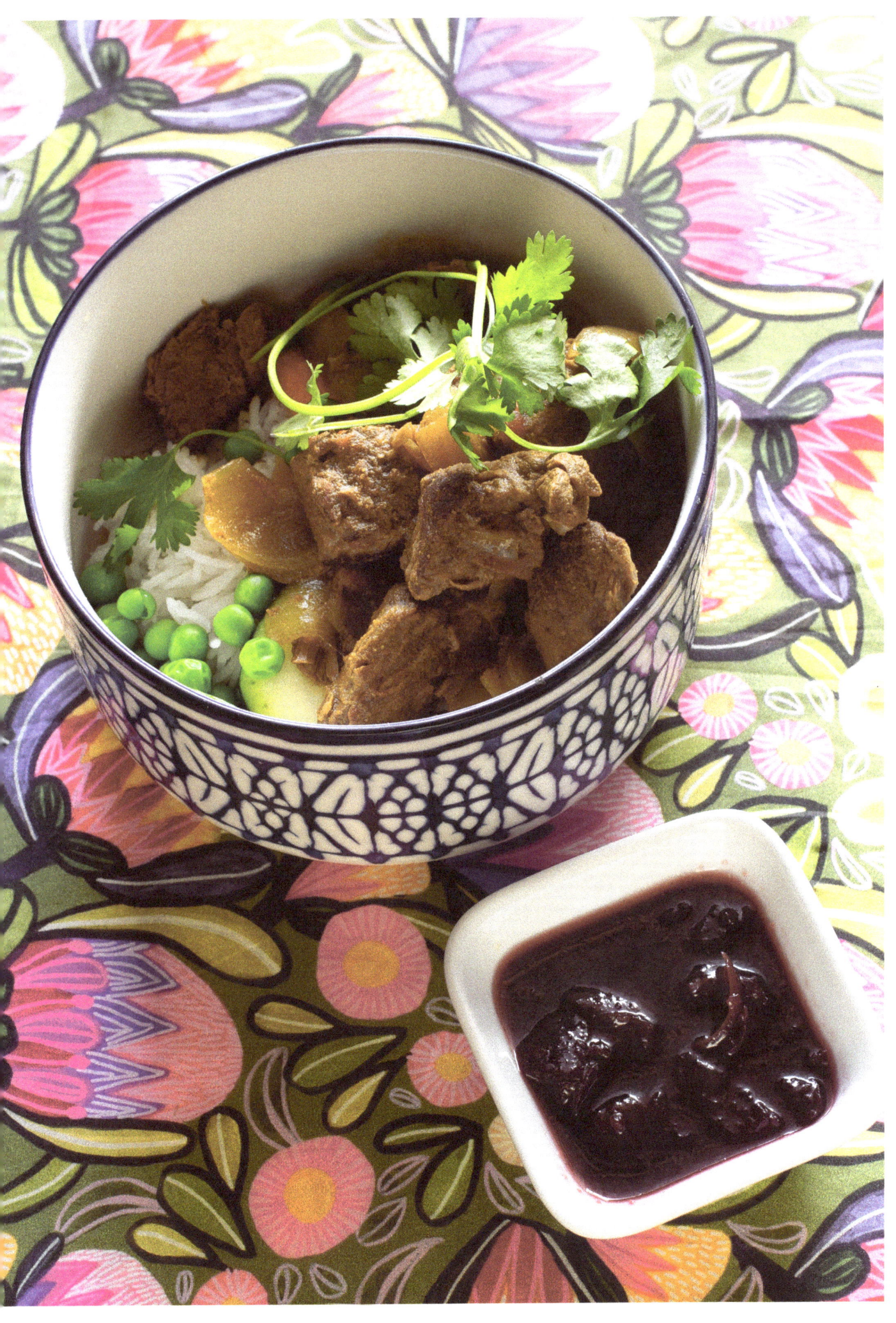

Lamb, Lentil and Tomato Soup

SERVES 6-8

about 700 grams lamb neck

1 onion (or equal from stock trimmings collected)

5 sprigs thyme

2 bay leaves

½ cup celery leaf

2 tablespoons flour

2 onions

1 tablespoon olive oil

3 cloves garlic

2 tablespoons oregano

1 tablespoon basil

2 carrots

2 sticks celery

500 grams tomatoes

½ cup lentils

1 cup pasta

1 cup peas

80 grams fetta

Roll the lamb neck in the flour and brown on all sides in a pan. Put in the slow cooker with two litres of water, the onion, bay leaf, celery leaf and cook on high for about 4 hours or until the meat is falling from the bone.

Soak the lentils overnight and cook until tender in boiling water, about 15 minutes. Cook the pasta in boiling water for about 10 minutes.

Dice the onion, carrot, celery and crush the garlic, sauté this in a large heavy base pot with the oil. Strain the stock into the pot with the sautéed vegetables and pull the meat off the neck and add this to the pot too.

Puree the tomatoes and add this to the pot, add the basil and oregano and simmer for 20 minutes then add the cooked lentils, pasta, peas and serve with the fetta crumbled on top.

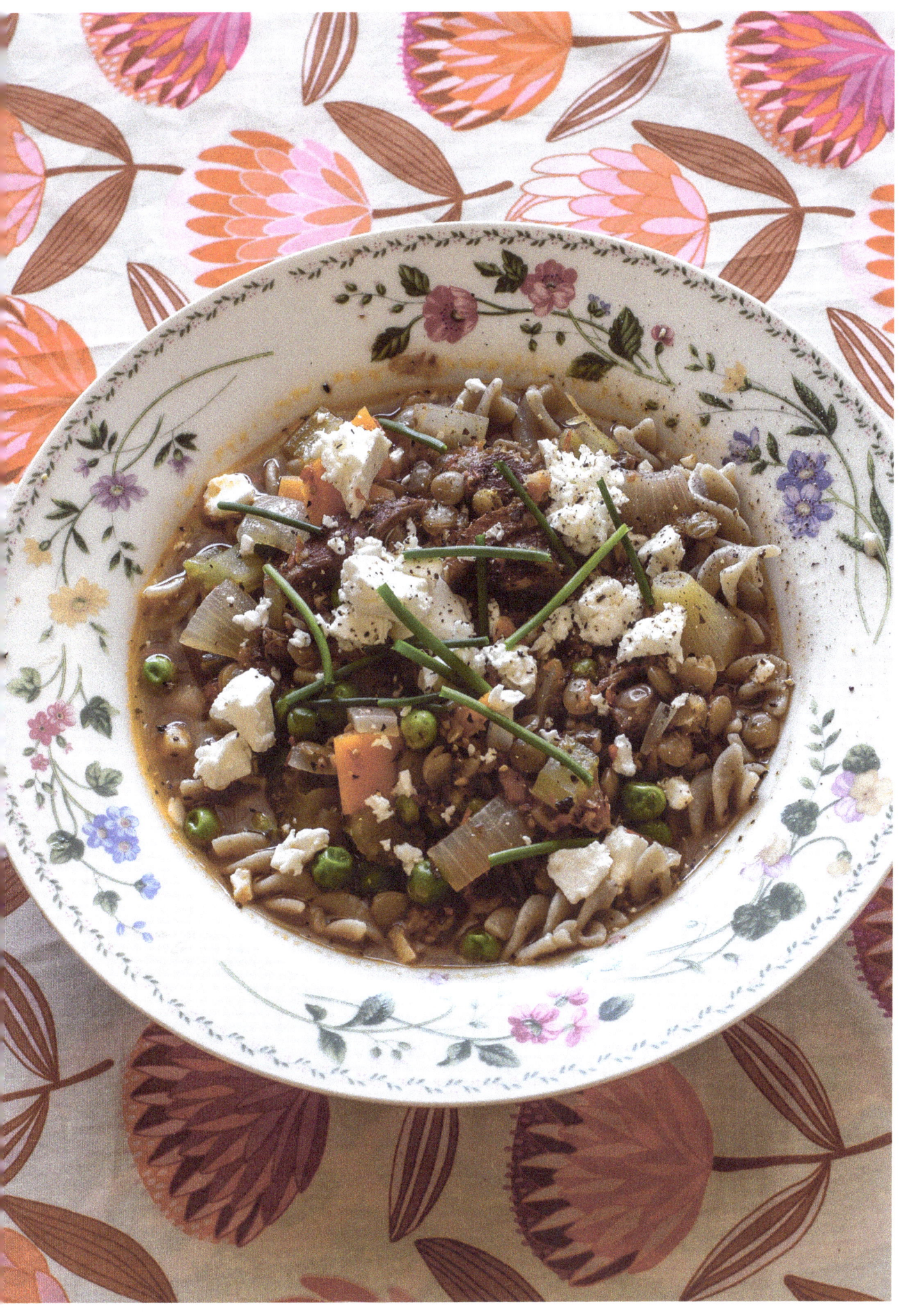

Cream of Broccoli and Bacon Soup

SERVES 4

Any veggie can be used in this soup, or a selection of veggies even the end of week veggie crisper clear out. Try a blue cheese for a fancier adult version.

1 onion

3 cloves garlic

3 rashers bacon

2 heads broccoli

3 tablespoons flour

1 litre vegetable or chicken stock

100ml cream

2 tablespoons tarragon

1 teaspoon thyme

100 grams cheese

salt and pepper

Dice onion, crush garlic and chop bacon and fry in a heavy based pot until soft and golden. Chop broccoli including stalk and add with the tarragon and thyme, add flour and cook for 2 minutes. Add stock, bring to a simmer and cook for about 20 minutes until broccoli is soft and cooked. Blend and add cream and cheese, bring back to the boil and season and serve.

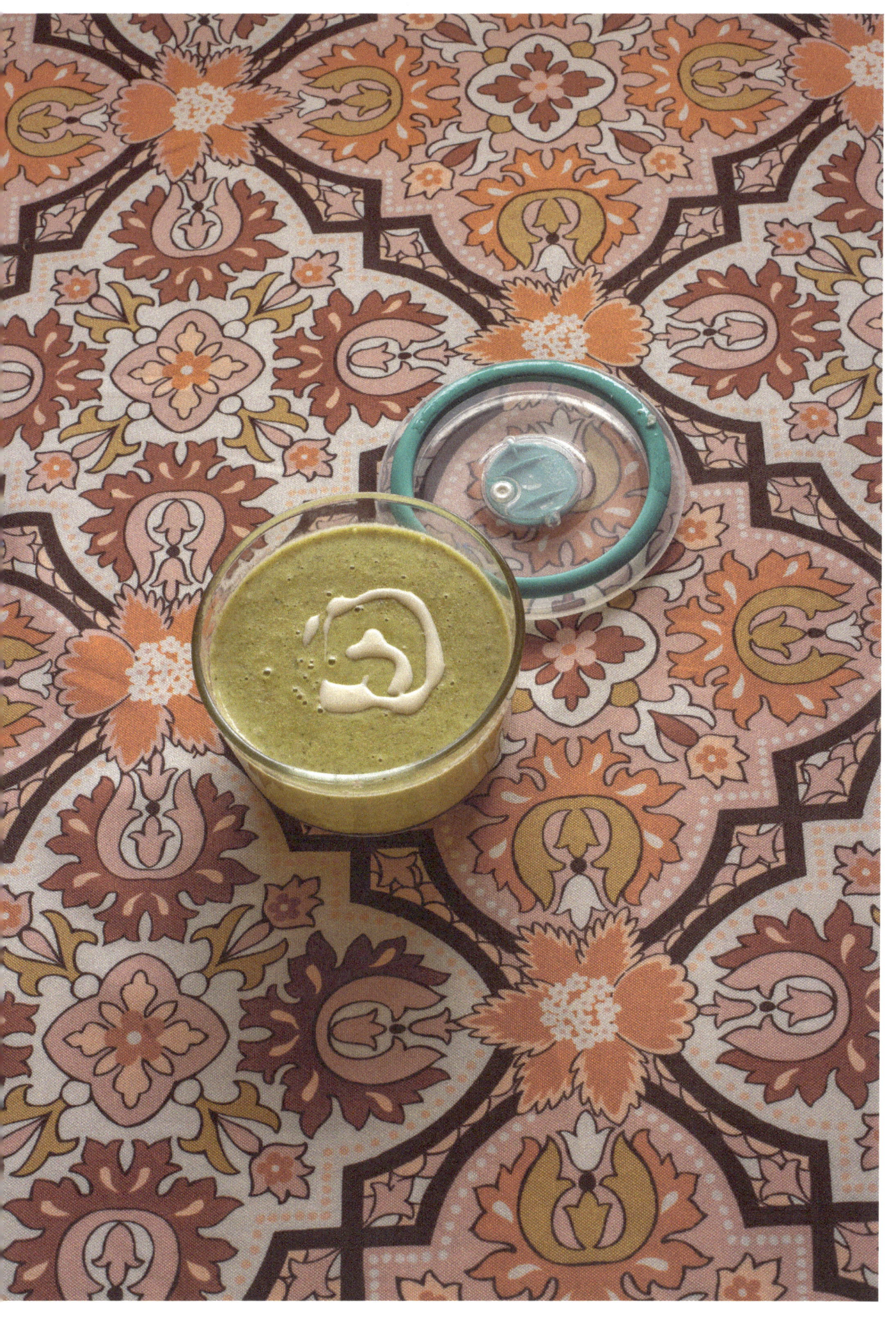

Fruit Leather

A fruit leather is simply cooked and pureed fruit, dried out. Simple and the kids love them. I don't add any sugar, you may want to depending on what fruit you are using. They should store for months on the shelf, it's a little bit more exciting way to preserve some of our apples from our tree and other fruits rather than bottling or stewing and freezing them! But it is after all just a dried fruit, so concentrated sugar, they are part of out treat consumption and they still get stuck in the teeth like the store bought variety, they may not have the additives and there are worse choices but whole fruit is better.

You can use any fruit to make them and they can be dried out in a food dehydrator or in the oven with the oven on about 90°C.

1- 2 kilo batches of fruits	In a pot or your thermocooker chop the apples and simmer until cooked, puree and spread onto a well-oiled tray about half a cm thick and dry in the oven for about 8 hours at 90°C or until completely dried out. You could use a food dehydrator if you have one.
	Store them between sheets of baking paper and then vacuumed packed in bags of 6 or wrapped and rolled up in an air tight jar ready to pop in the lunch box

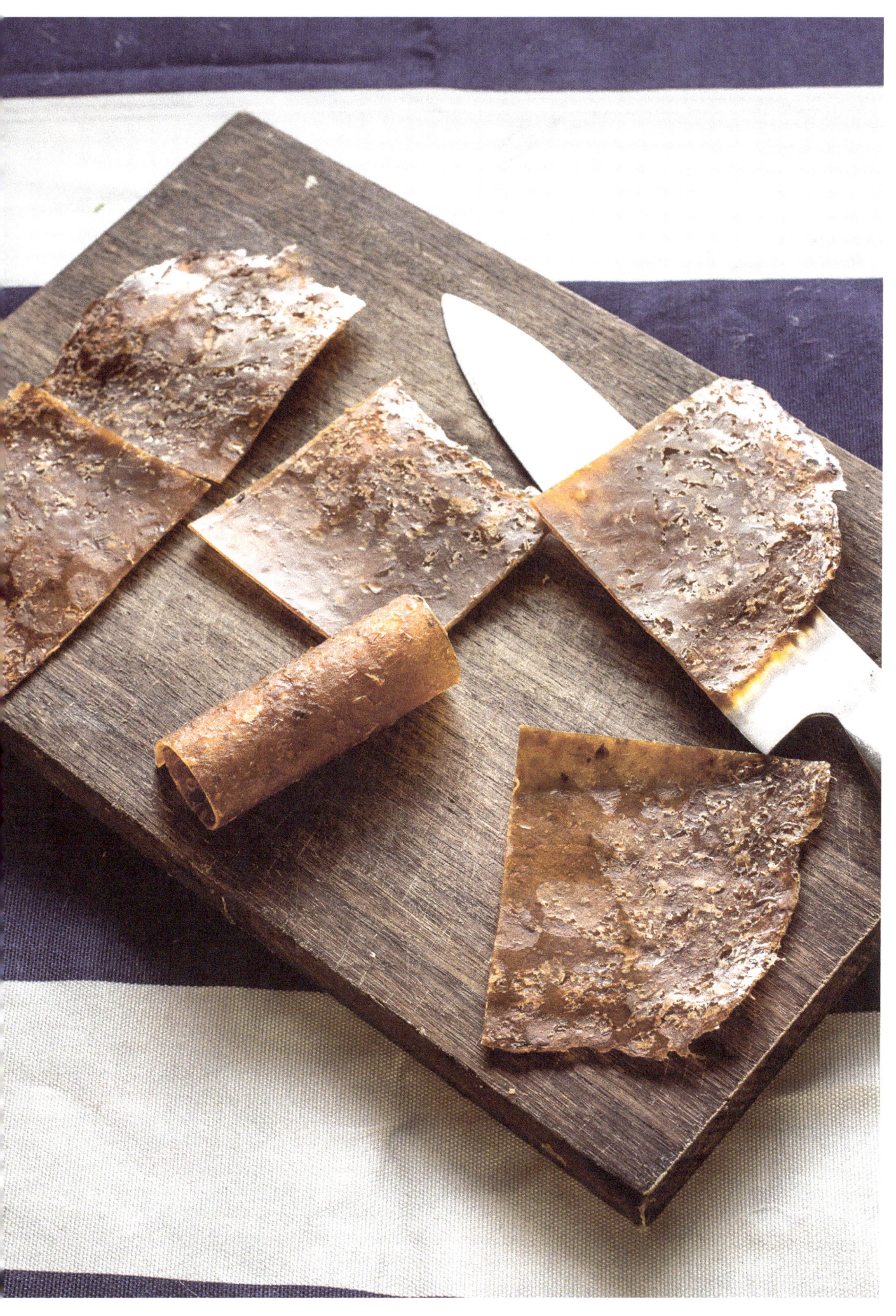

Honey and Mustard Slow Cooked Beef with Thyme Polenta

SERVES 4-6

You can use any of the stewing steak cuts like oyster blade, chuck or blade. This beef is also delicious in a wrap with broccoli salad (see page 38).

800 grams beef

1 tablespoon flour

2 onions

2 cloves garlic

3 large carrots

1 stick celery

1 leek

¼ cup balsamic vinegar

3 bay leaves

6 big sprigs thyme

2 tablespoons Dijon mustard

2 tablespoons honey

400 grams crushed tomatoes

400 grams beef stock salt and pepper

Cut the beef into a chunky dice before rolling in the flour and browning it in a pan over a medium heat with a little oil. Put the beef in a slow cooker with the crushed garlic, peeled and chunky chopped onion and carrot, chopped celery and leek and all the other ingredients. Give it a good mix and cook on low for about 6 hours or until falling apart. Serve with veggies and mashed potato, cous cous or polenta.

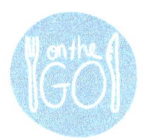

Packs well in a thermos but put the polenta on top. Or pack the broccoli salad and the beef In the thermos.

Thyme Polenta

SERVES 4-6

2 cloves garlic

½ brown onion

dash olive oil

500ml milk

100 grams polenta

10 large sprigs thyme

40 grams parmesan salt and pepper

Crush the garlic and finely chop the onion and sauté in the olive oil in a heavy based pot. Add milk and bring back to a simmer while continually stirring. Add the thyme and polenta and continue stirring for 15-20 minutes until the polenta is cooked and thick, add cheese and season. You can do all this with ease in the thermocooker.

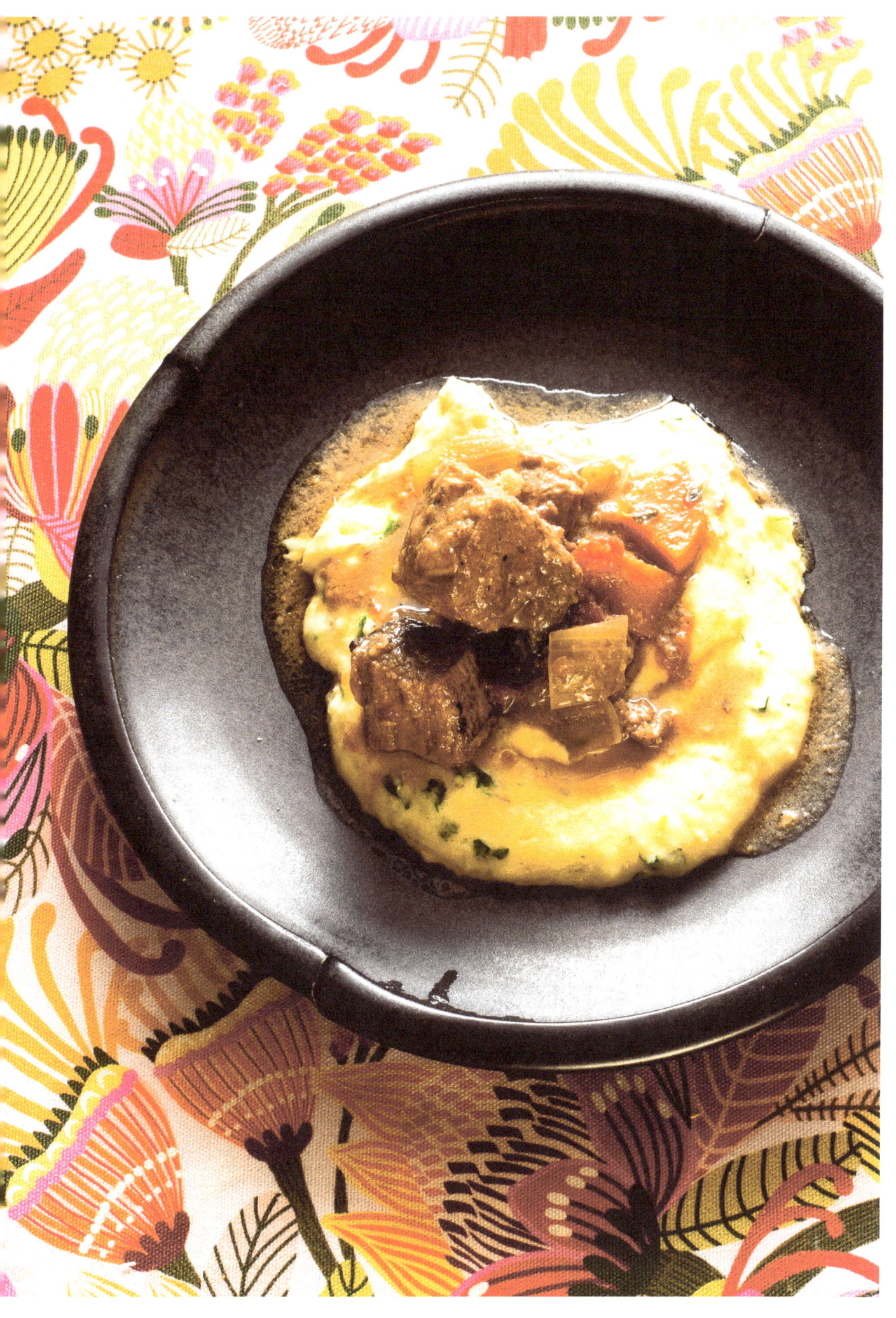

Pumpkin, Mushroom and Chicken Risotto

SERVES 4-6

There are so many different ideas for risotto such as beetroot and goats cheese, bacon or other smoked meats, seafood, salmon, and loads of different veggies like asparagus, fennel, and herbs can go in for flavour and gut health and diversity. However I find I just need to keep an eye on my rice to vegetable/meat ratio so it is not just eating a bowl of nutrient- limited rice. If you have a thermocooker you will know how to make this in it.

1 tablespoon olive oil

1 medium brown onion

3 cloves garlic

150 grams mushrooms

500 grams chicken

300 grams pumpkin

200 grams aborio rice

600ml chicken stock

2 cups spinach leaves

50 grams parmesan

50ml cream

1 tablespoon basil

1 tablespoon oregano

2 cups peas

salt and pepper

Crush garlic and dice onion and sauté in the oil in a large heavy based pot, slice mushrooms and rice add to the pot and sauté for a further minute, and stock and simmer.

Add diced pumpkin and chicken and simmer gently continuously stirring for about 15-20 minutes until rice and pumpkin is cooked.

Add cream, cheese spinach, peas until heated through and season with salt and pepper

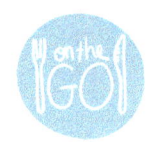

Surprisingly, a cooked risotto actually freezes really well so make extra to freeze in lunch portions to defrost and pop in the thermos for a quick and satisfying packed lunch in the thermos.

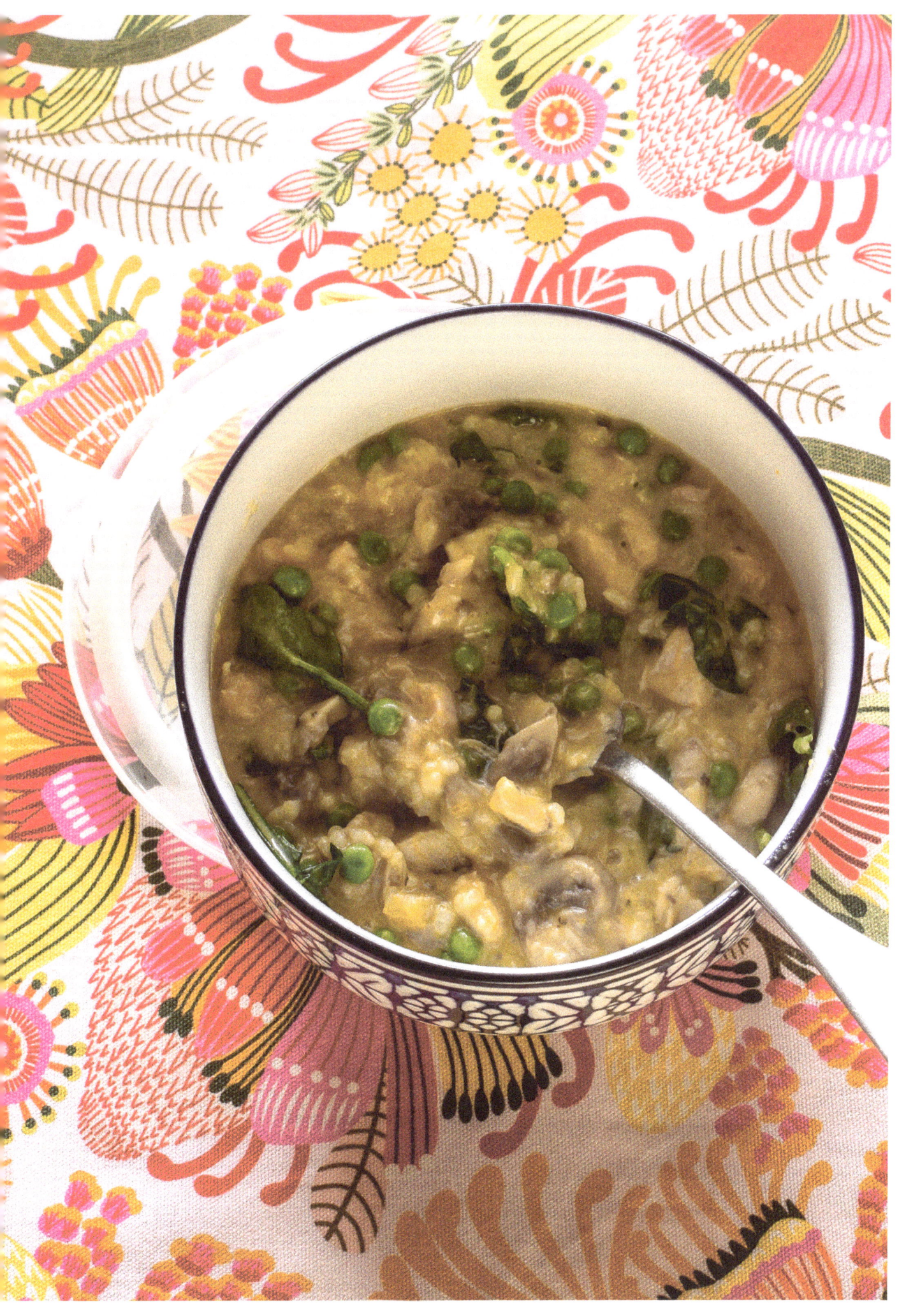

Slow Cooked Lamb, Silver Beet and Fetta Cannelloni

SERVES 4

Silky handmade pasta and slow cooked meat is a gorgeous combo. This dish is fancy enough for a dinner party but just because dinner is eaten in the carpark at the kids activities from a thermos does not mean it has to be boring! And this can be prepared ahead.

1 tablespoon flour

700 grams lamb chops

1 onion

3 cloves garlic

1 tablespoon basil

1 tablespoon oregano

1 pinch salt and pepper

400 grams tomatoes

1 teaspoon rosemary

1 teaspoon thyme

2 cups pumpkin

1 cup silver beet

100 grams fetta

100 grams cheddar

PASTA

2 large eggs

150-200 grams plain flour

Roll the chops in the flour and brown in a pan on the stove then transfer them to the slow cooker. Peel and dice the onion, crush the garlic and chop the herbs and tomatoes and put this all in the slow cooker, add a good pinch of salt and pepper and cook on low for 5 ½ hours or until the meat is falling off the bone. Put it in another container in the fridge to cool down. When cool remove the fat from the top and discard. Remove the bones and discard.

Roast the pumpkin by chopping it into a 2cm dice and rolling in olive oil and laying it in a baking dish and baking for about 25 minutes until cooked.

Separate most of the sauce from the meat and put this sauce aside. This will be your sauce for the top of the cannelloni, it does not matter if there are a few bits of meat still in it.

Shred the silver beet and mix this with the cheeses, cooled roast pumpkin and the meat to make the filling.

To make the pasta, either in the food processor or a bowl mix the egg into 150 grams flour and knead well, this dough might be still wet and need more flour. When it is a firm dough, roll out on the pasta machine starting at the widest setting and then lower the setting after each roll through until the pasta is thin sheets, cut into 15cm long sheets. Cook for about 3 minutes in boiling water and cool.

Lay the filling in the middle of each sheet and roll, lay in a baking tray and top with the sauce and parmesan cheese. Bake for about 25 minutes in a moderate (180°C) oven.

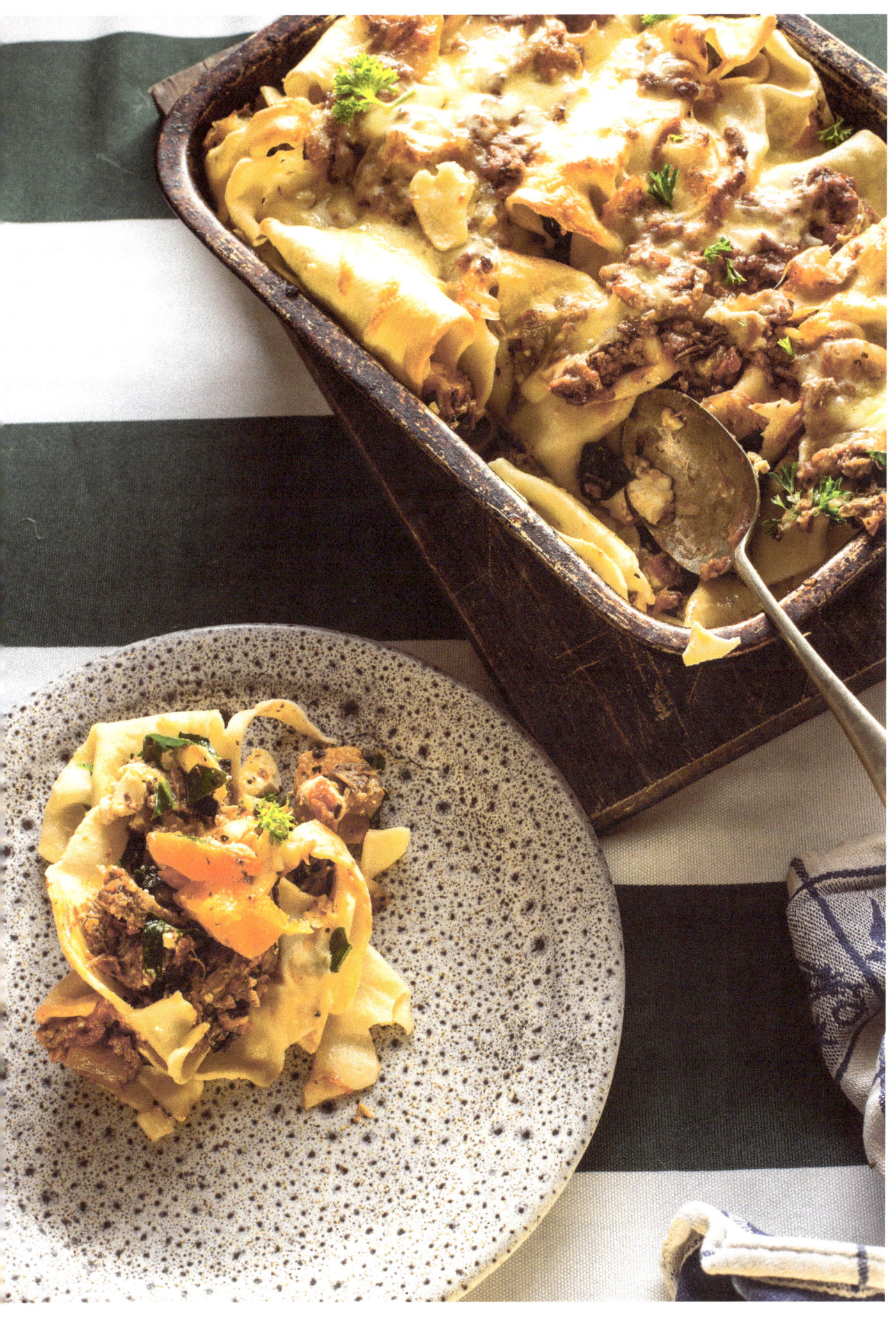

Honey Soy Brown Rice Salad & Tassal Cooked Tassie Salmon (Naturally Smoked)

SERVES 4-6

You can use whatever veggies you like in this salad and if you have salmon in the freezer this meal can be pulled together from food in the pantry like I have included here as an example, handy for the day before shopping! This is one of my favourite pack before 6am to eat at 6pm dinners as it stores well in a cooler bag with a few icepacks all day. The same salad is delicious with chicken.

DRESSING

3 tablespoons extra virgin olive oil

2 tablespoons white vinegar

1 tablespoon honey

1 tablespoon soy

¼ teaspoon sea salt

¼ teaspoon pepper

SALAD

2 cups brown rice cooked in stock (page 29)

1 cup peas

1 cup corn

1 tin white beans

1 small head broccoli

1 cup cabbage

2 cups spinach leaves

500 grams Tassal Cooked Tassie Salmon (Naturally smoked)

To make the dressing find a large bowl and mix all the dressing ingredients together.

Add the rice, chopped broccoli, sliced cabbage, peas, corn, beans and mix well. Add the spinach and salmon just before serving but if it's a meal-to-go, pop them on top in the storage container and mix through before eating so the leaves do not wilt.

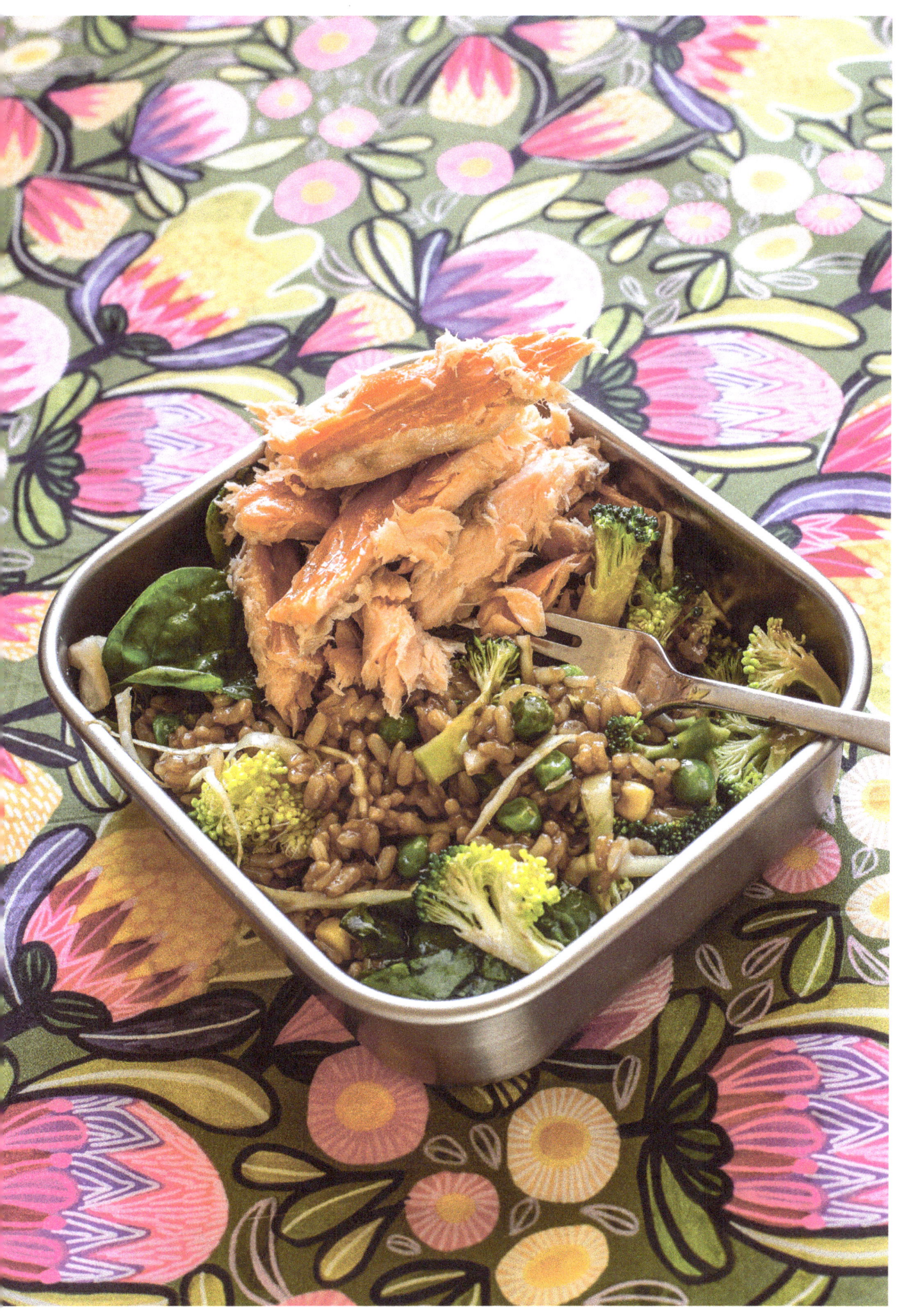

Apricot Chicken and Sage Buttered Cous Cous

SERVES 4

8 chicken legs

2 tablespoons flour

1 small onion

2 cloves garlic

100ml stock

1 teaspoon thyme

1 teaspoon sage

½ teaspoon cumin

pinch pepper

2 cups apricots

COUS COUS

2 cups chicken stock

2 cups cous cous

1 tablespoon butter

1 clove garlic

1 tablespoon sage

1 tablespoon thyme

pinch pepper

steamed greens to serve

To cook the chicken, roll the chicken in the flour, and over a medium heat in a pan brown the legs on all sides. Put the chicken in the bottom of the slow cooker with the onion, crushed garlic, chopped thyme and sage, cumin, pepper, apricots and stock, cook on high for about four hours or until the meat is falling off the bone.

To cook the cous cous bring the stock to the boil and add the cous cous and cover for about 3 minutes. Melt the butter in a pan and add the crushed garlic and sauté, the butter will froth, toss through the herbs and pepper and mix this through the cous cous and serve with some steamed greens.

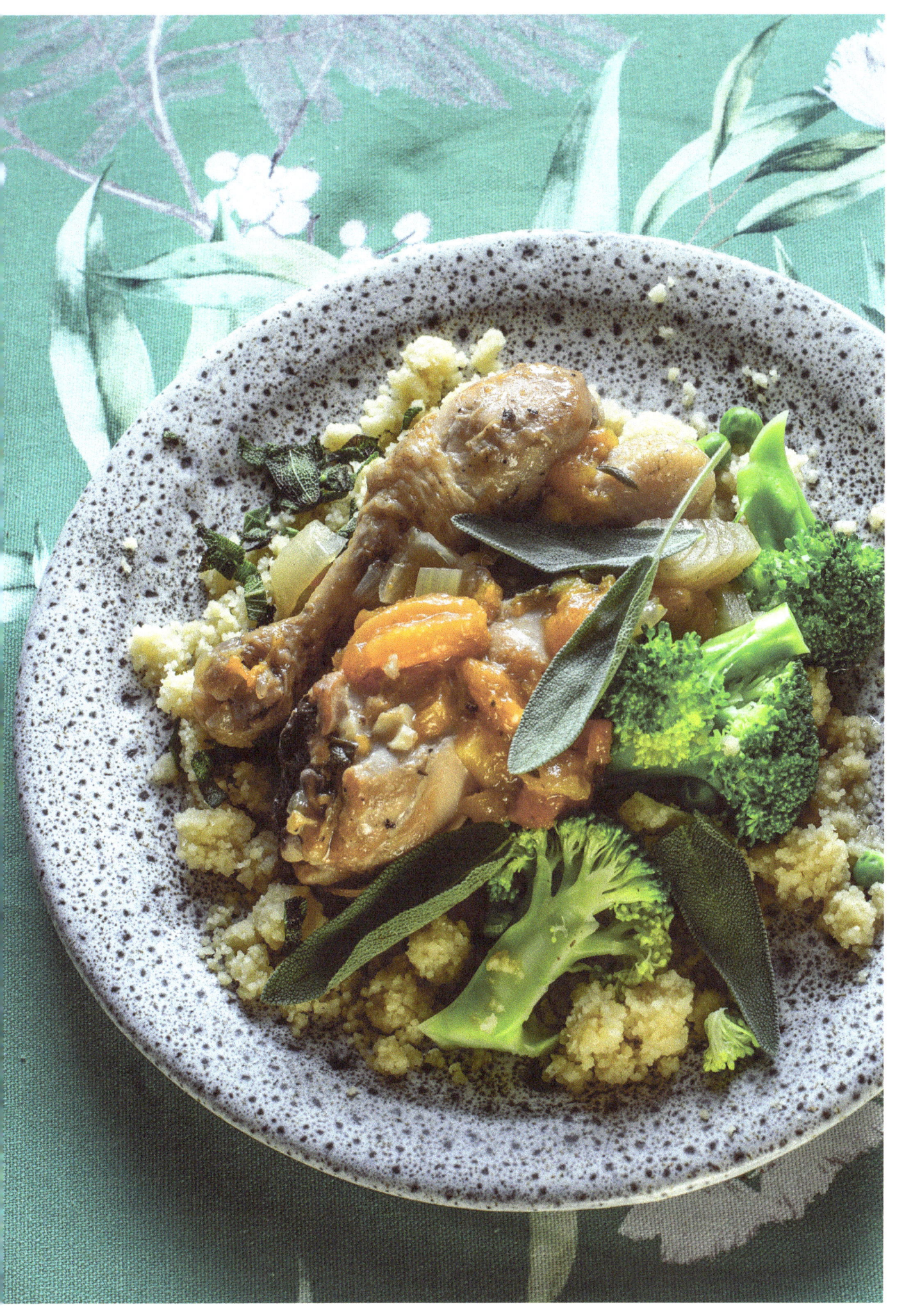

Slow-Cooker Roast Lamb and Cous Cous Salad

SERVES 4-6

This salad is made from pretty much whatever I have in the pantry/fridge and it changes each time I make it! You could use tinned beans, chickpeas, cucumber, fetta, grilled haloumi or other cheese, grilled veggies such as zucchini or capsicum, olives, sundried tomatoes, balsamic or red wine vinegar. I make it with cold leftover roast lamb for lunch with leftover roast veggies in the salad or as the main meal with lamb cooked especially for the salad.

1 cup cous cous

1 cup stock

1 teaspoon butter

1 teaspoon preserved lemon

1 cup roast pumpkin (roast extra with your lamb)

600 grams roast lamb

2 large tomatoes

1 cup peas

1 cup lettuce

20 mint leaves

20 chives

1 tablespoon extra virgin olive oil

2 cloves garlic

80 grams fetta cheese

salt and pepper

tzatziki (page 60)

To cook the cous cous, bring the stock to the boil add the cous cous and cover for 5 minutes, then fold in the butter and cool.

Crush the garlic, dunk the peas in boiling water for a minute and strain, chop all the other ingredients, and toss together and serve.

Mid week meal hint: Have you tried your roast lamb in the slow cooker? I like my leisurely Sunday lamb roast roasted in the oven with all the veggies but the slow-cooker is handy set on a timer to start for the midweek meal. Cut a garlic bulb in half through the middle and put in the bottom of the slow cooker and slice an onion, put lamb on top with a handful of rosemary and thyme, sprinkle with salt and pepper and cook in the slow cooker for about 6 hours and the meat falls of the bone.

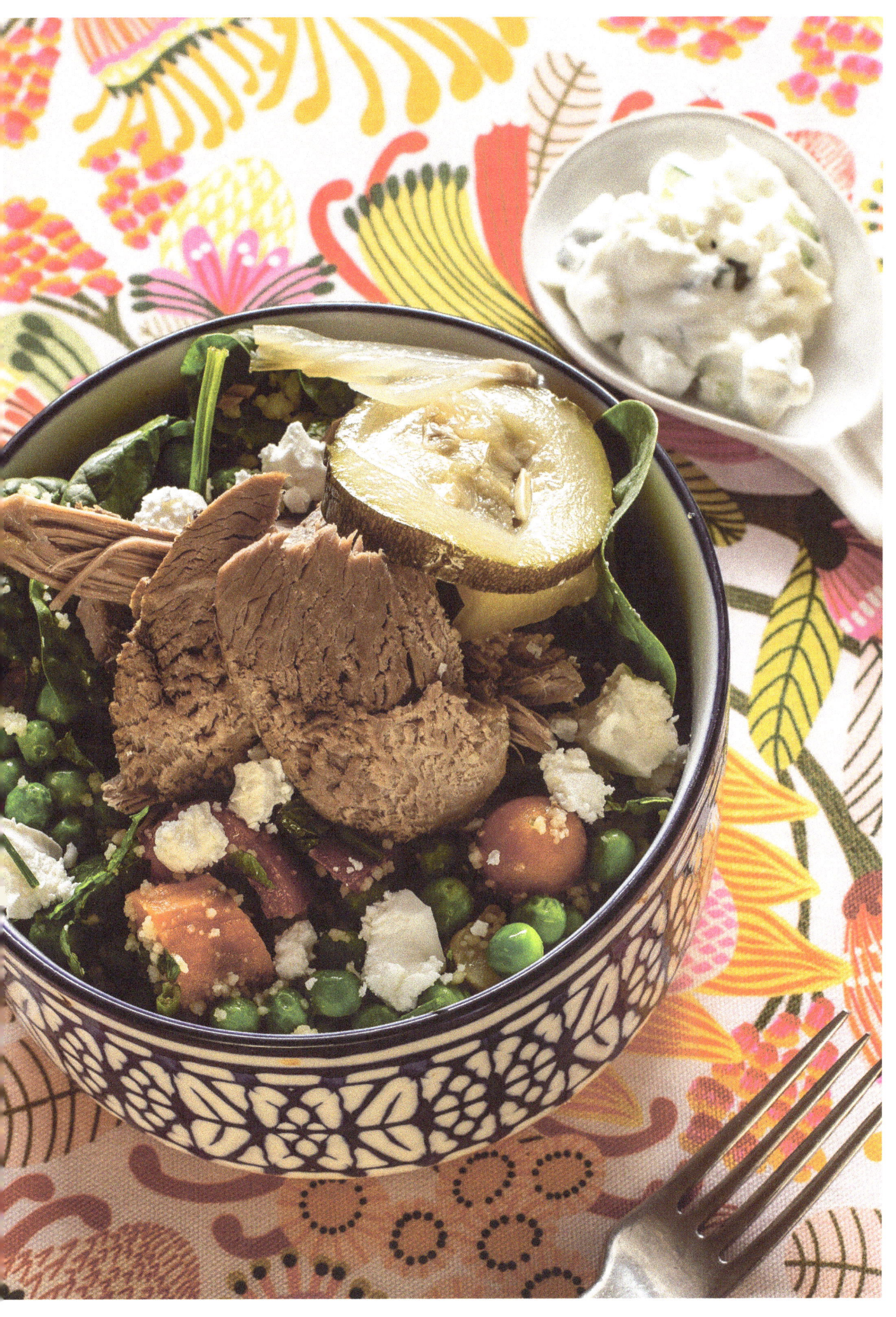

Green Peppered Chicken Liver Pate

MAKES 4 SMALL POTS

1 tablespoon butter

500 grams chicken livers

½ to 1 tablespoons green peppercorns

1 rasher bacon

1 small onion

1 clove garlic

1 teaspoon dried basil

½ teaspoon dried thyme

100ml cream

sea salt

extra virgin olive oil to top and store

In a heavy based pan or your thermocooker, sauté the butter, chopped bacon, peeled and chopped onion, peeled and chopped garlic and sauté until soft and fragrant.

Add the livers, peppercorns and herbs and sauté over a low heat until just cooked. Add the cream and bring to the boil.

Purée and place in pots, top with a thin layer of extra virgin olive oil to set in the refrigerator.

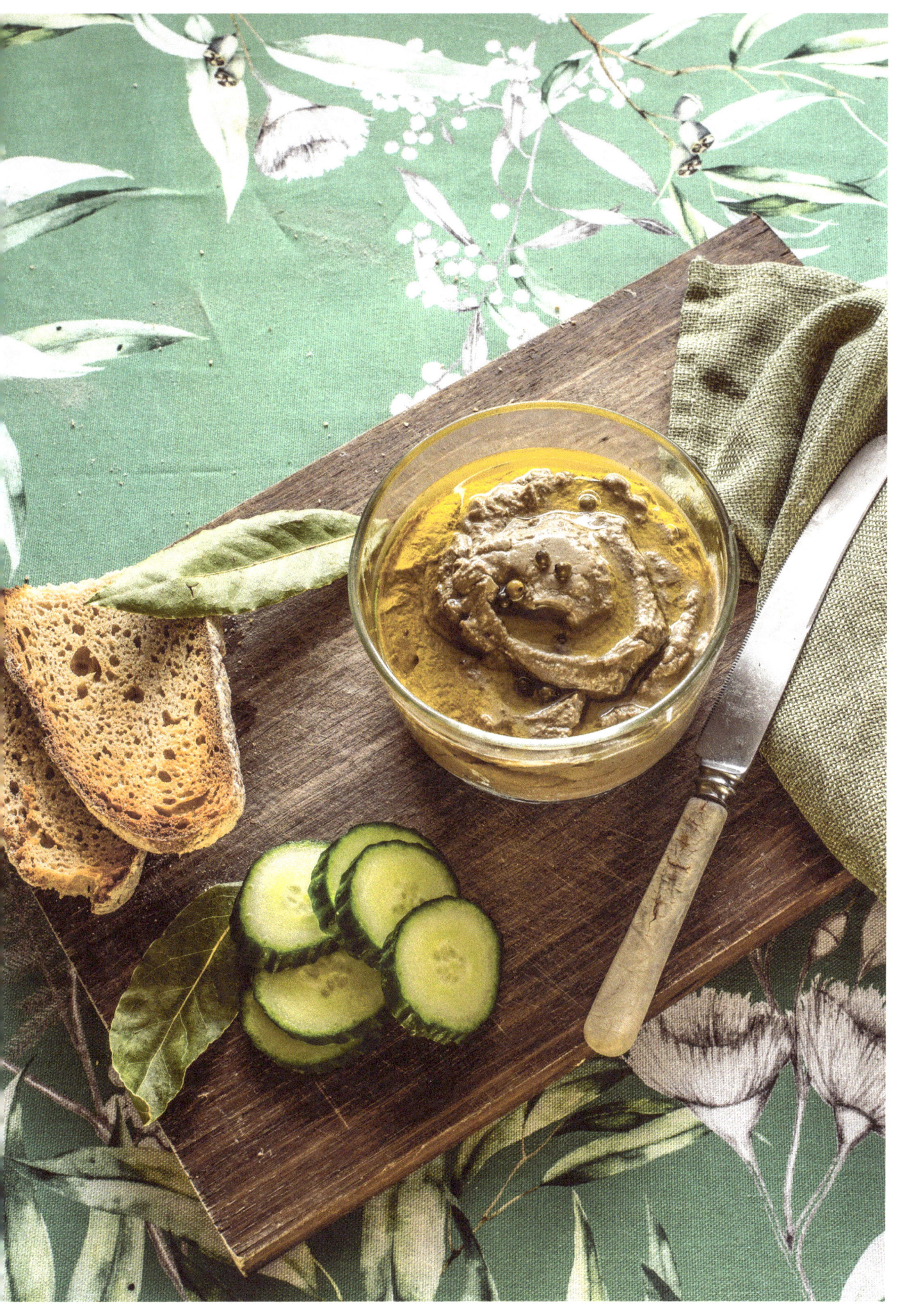

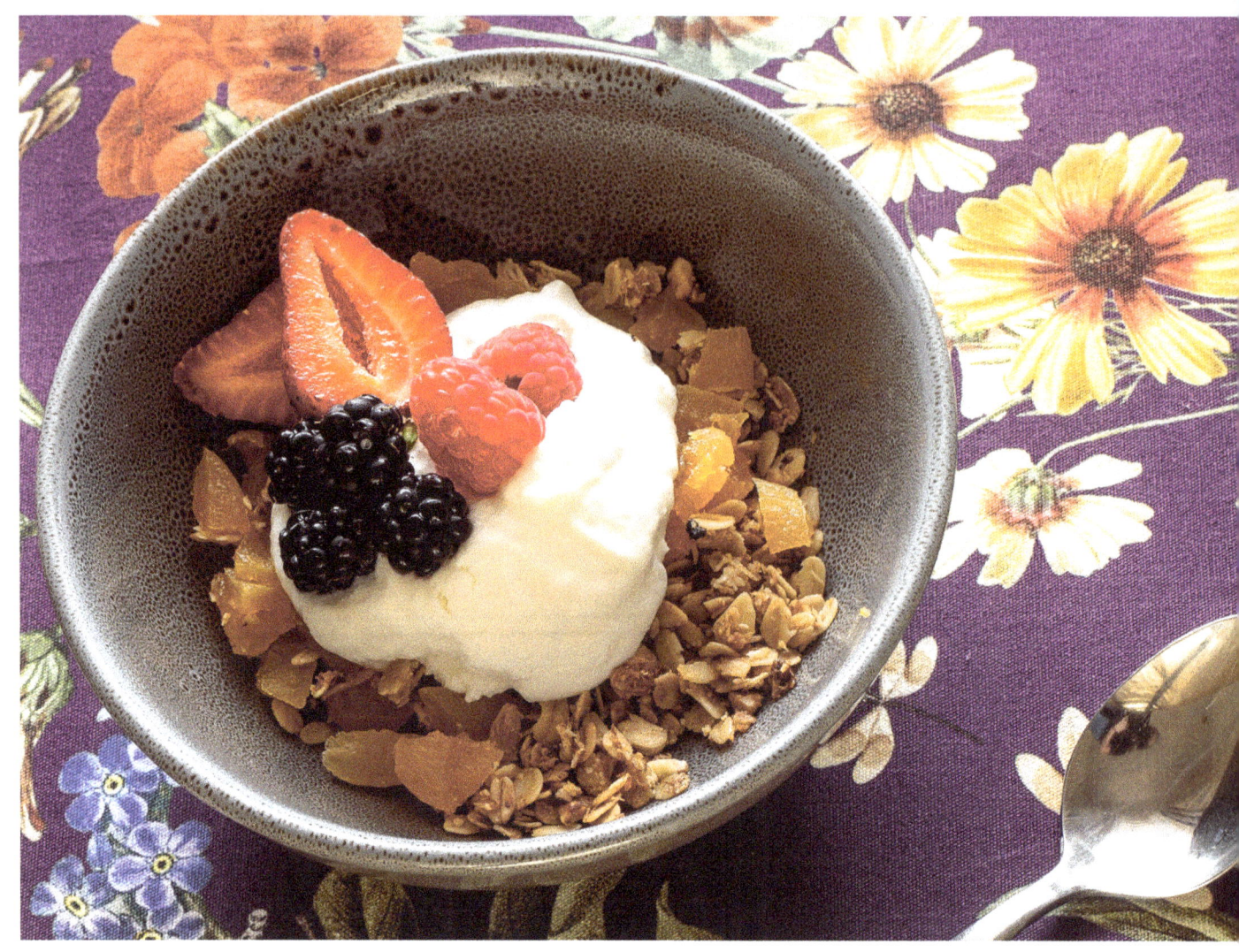

Apricot and Almond Toasted Muesli

MAKES ONE BIG JAR ENOUGH FOR 12 OR MORE BREAKFASTS

There are many different flavour combinations you can use. Find a gorgeous Campo de Flori Lavender and honey toasted muesli recipe in Tasmania Pantry 2. This makes a quick dessert and after school snack too.

100ml delicate or medium extra virgin olive oil

3 tablespoons honey

4 cups rolled oats

½ cup desiccated coconut

1 teaspoon cinnamon

1 cup almonds slithered

2 cups apricot dried

milk or yogurt to serve

Heat the oven to 170°C.

Mix together the oats, nuts and desiccated coconut. Warm the oil and honey in a saucepan on the stove. Pour the syrup mixture into the oat mixture and mix well.

Divide the mixture on to 2 large baking dishes and bake, stirring every 5 minutes for 20 minutes until golden. Cool then stir through the dried apricots.

Serve with milk or yogurt for breakfast.

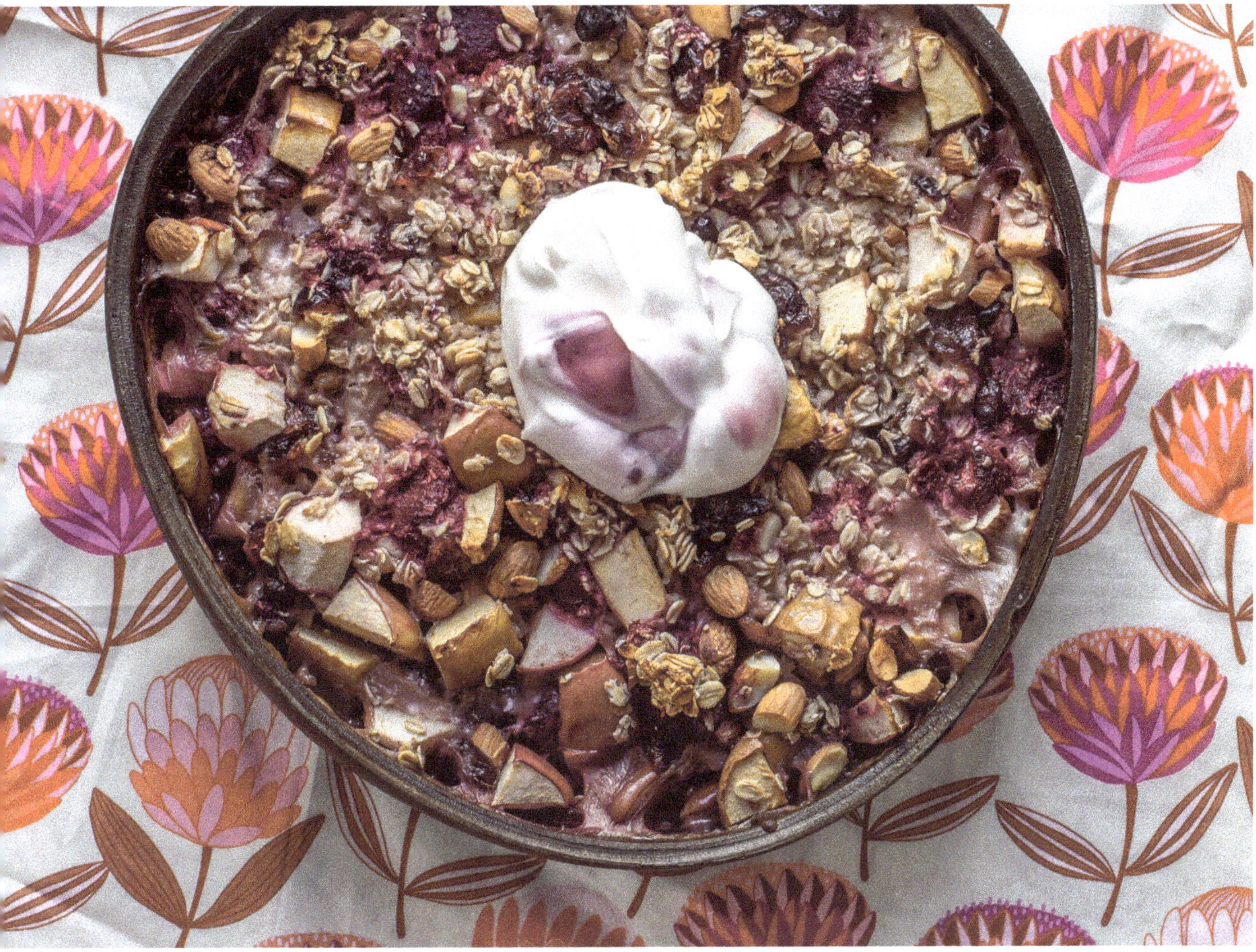

Baked Hazelnut, Pear, Berry and Cinnamon Porridge

SERVES 6

This can be baked with chunks of whole seasonal fruits for a delicious easy to serve breakfast. Or you can use any frozen or preserved fruits and ideas of fruit and nut combinations. Try Campo De Flori or Port Arthur Lavender, honey, vanilla and cinnamon for extra flavour.

2 cups milk

1 cup oats

1 tablespoon honey

1 teaspoon cinnamon

½ cup hazelnuts

3 pears

1 cup berries

1 cup almonds

1 teaspoon vanilla

Heat the oven to 180°C.

Chop the pears of the core and chop into a rough cm dice, place in a casserole dish with the milk, water, oats, honey, cinnamon, berries and hazelnuts. Mix well and place in the oven to bake for around 30 minutes to cook.

Yogurt to serve

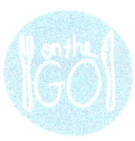

Pop in the oven first thing in the morning to scoop into bowls or the thermos to eat when you get a chance to chew and enjoy!!

Packed - *Nutrient dense food for on the go lifestyles*

Smoothie and Smoothie Bowls Ideas

SERVES 1

Thrown in the blender, and consumed on the way to school or work, smoothies are too easy, and packed full of nutrition. A quick and handy after school snack too! Smoothie bowls are just a prettier way to serve them with fruits decorations on top. You can use any combination of fresh frozen fruits and vegetables but just make sure to get some protein in with eggs, nuts and yogurt to keep those bellies full longer. There is a risk with eating raw eggs (AND IT IS A VERY SMALL RISK) of salmonella but that's one I am prepared to take. I make all my own mayo and aioli with raw eggs and have so far avoided and infection.

1 egg

2 tablespoons natural yogurt

½ cup milk

100 gram frozen berries

½ teaspoon honey

½ teaspoon vanilla essence

OTHER INGREDIENT IDEAS

oats

nuts

chia seeds

pumpkin seeds

peanut butter

quinoa

cocoa nibs

Banana

cacao

hemp seeds

any frozen, preserved, tinned or fresh seasonal fruits

spinach

Campo De flori lavender

Port Arthur Lavender

To make a Smoothie throw all the ingredients in a blender or thermocooker and blend to desired consistency.

For Smoothie Bowl pour into a bowl and decorate the top with sliced fruits and seeds.

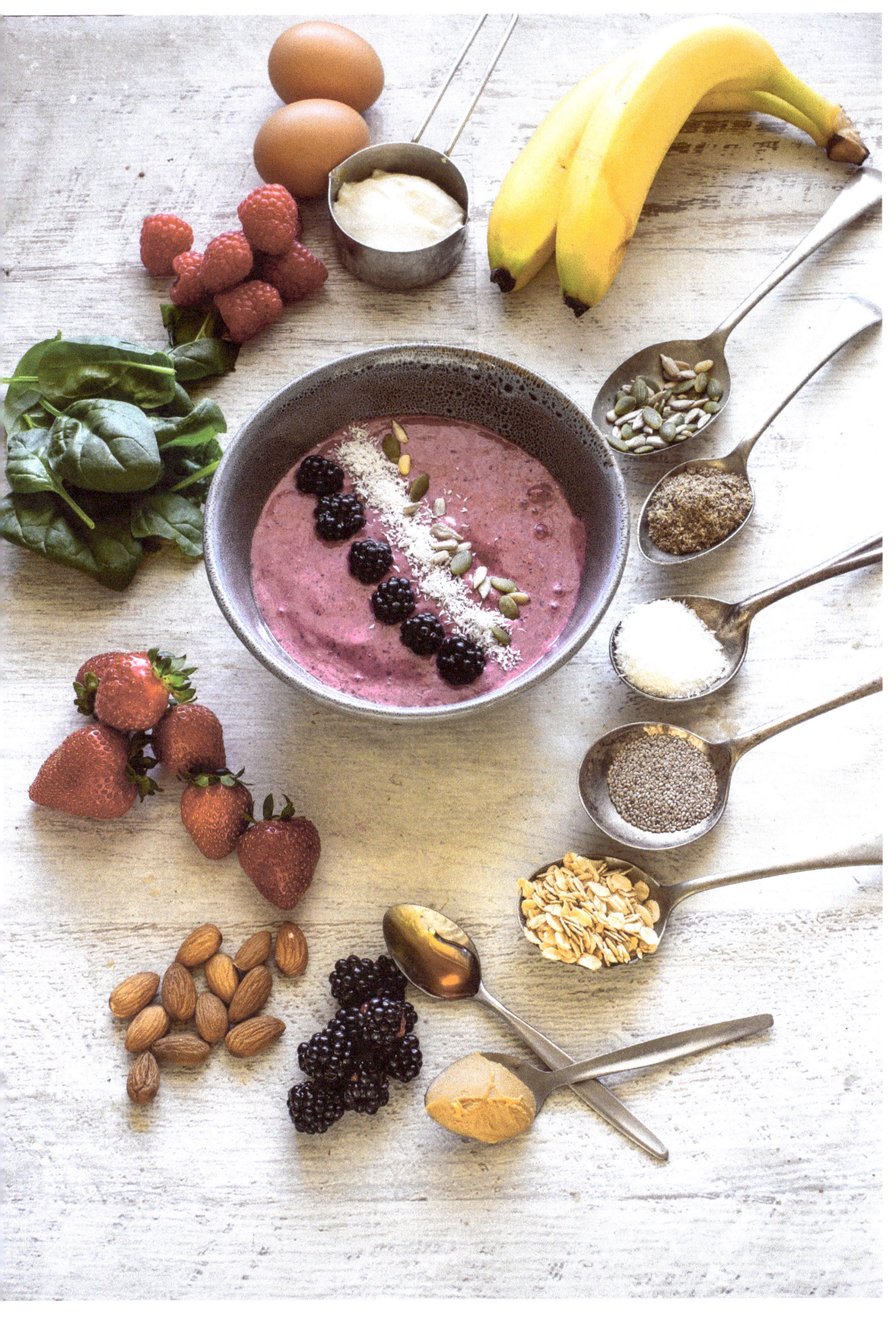

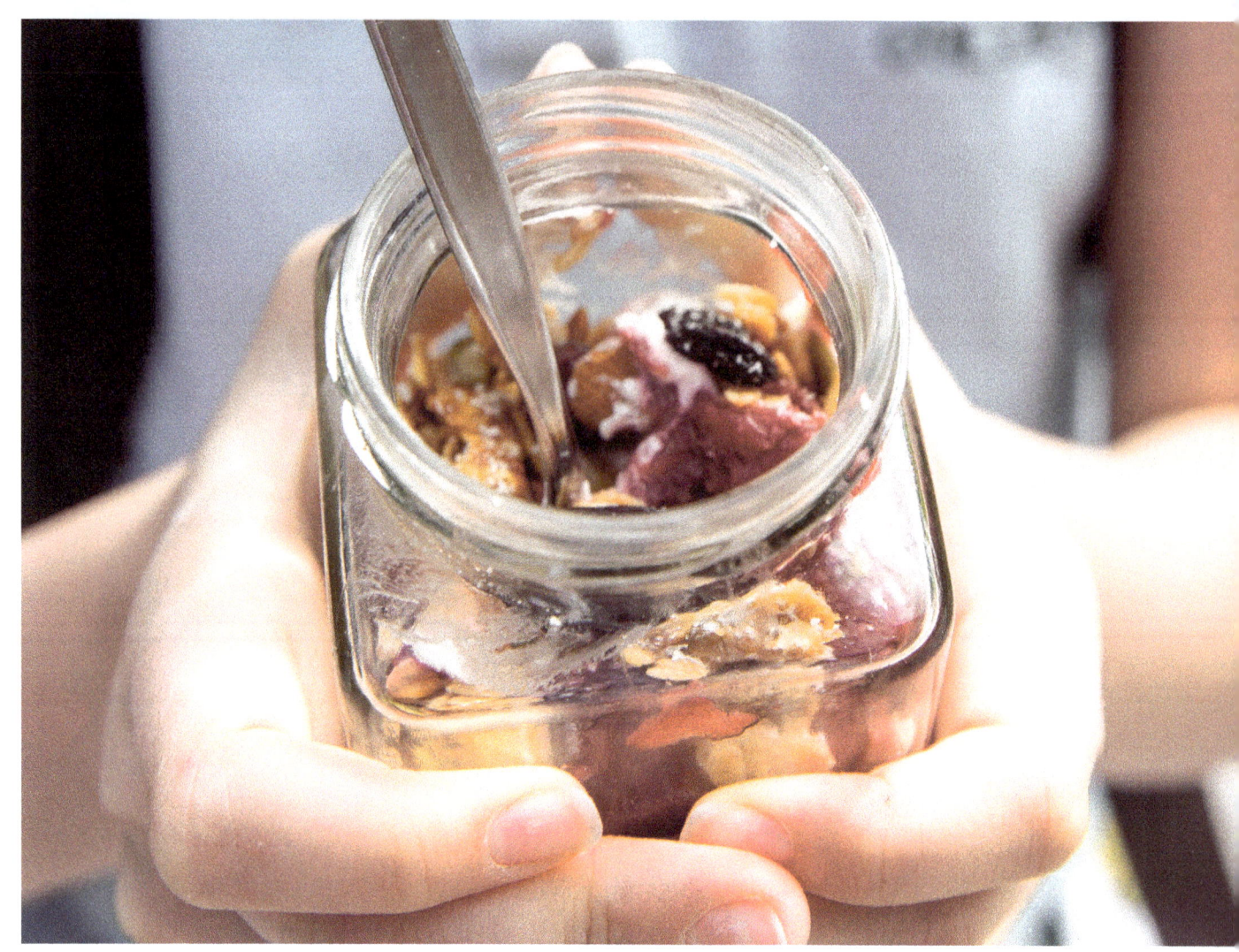

Breakfast Trifle

SERVES 4

Find my homemade vanilla yogurt recipe on my website

1 ½ cups rolled oats

⅔ cup apple juice

1 tablespoon sultanas

1 teaspoon dried pumpkin seeds

1 teaspoon almond flakes

1 grated apple

600ml yogurt

2 punnets berries

To make the bircher muesli, grate the apple into a bowl and mix with the oats, juice, sultanas, seeds and almonds. Refrigerate overnight.

Serve the muesli layered with the yogurt and fresh berries.

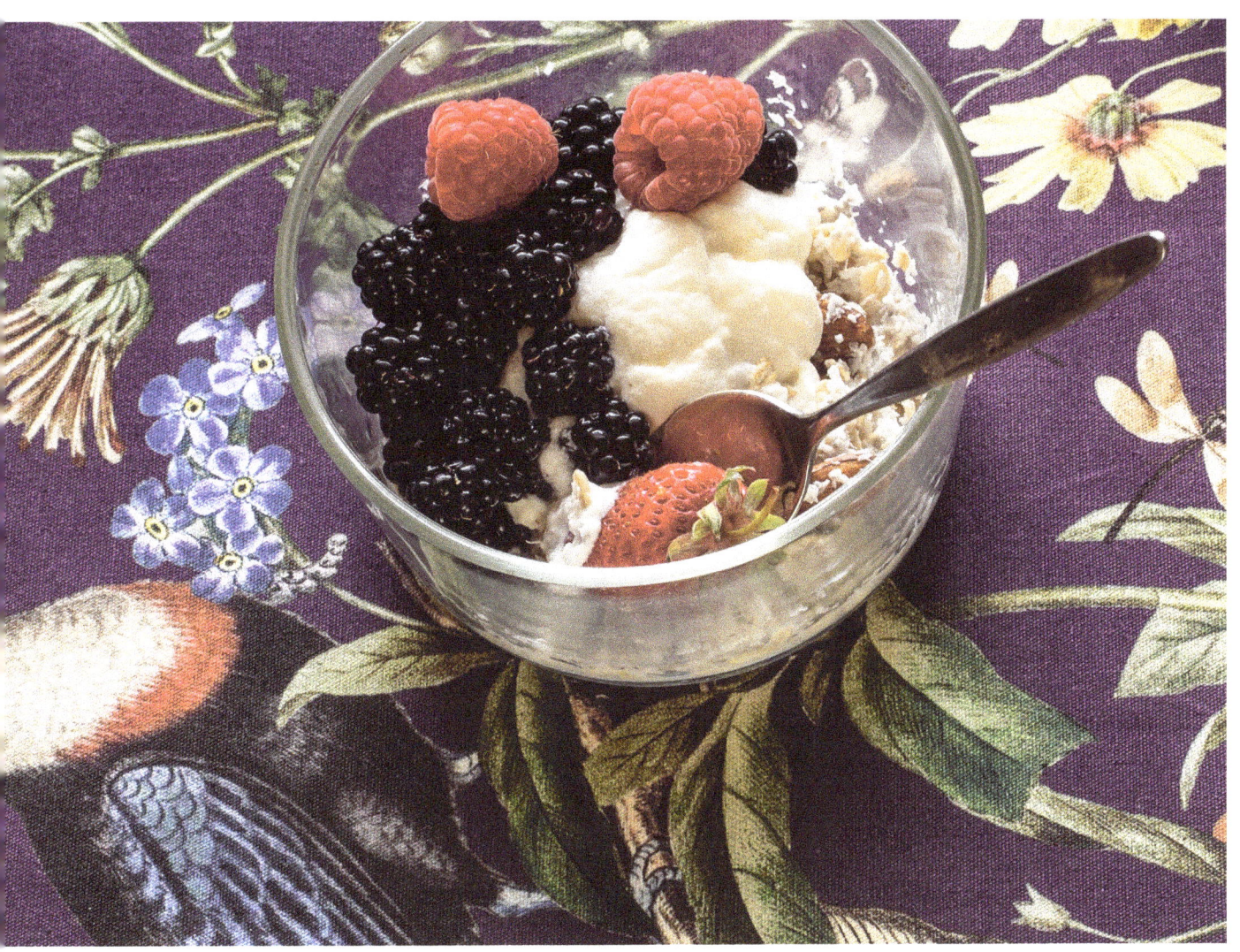

Berry, Apple Overnight Oats

SERVES 4-6 FOR BREAKFAST OR SNACK

There are some more great overnight oat ideas in my book 'The Tasmania Pantry 2' and loads of different fruits, nuts and seed combinations can be used. It is a great breakfast to prepare the night before a busy morning for a grab and go breakfast.

1 cup oats

2 apples

1 cup milk

1 teaspoon honey

½ cup yogurt

2 tablespoons almonds

1 tablespoon coconut

TO SERVE

1 cup berries

Grate the apples and mix with the oats, milk, honey, yogurt, almonds and coconut and refrigerate overnight. Top with berries and serve.

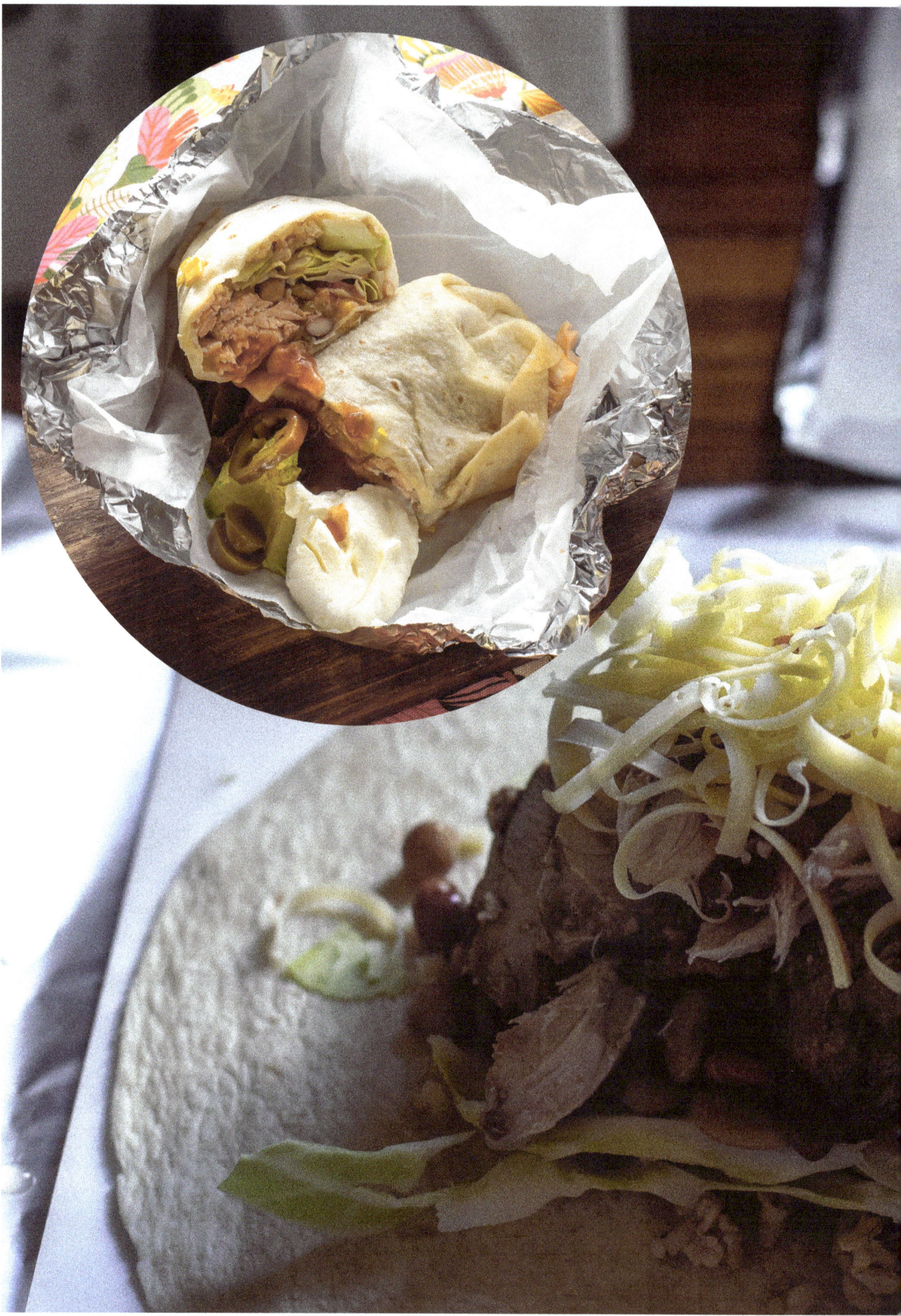

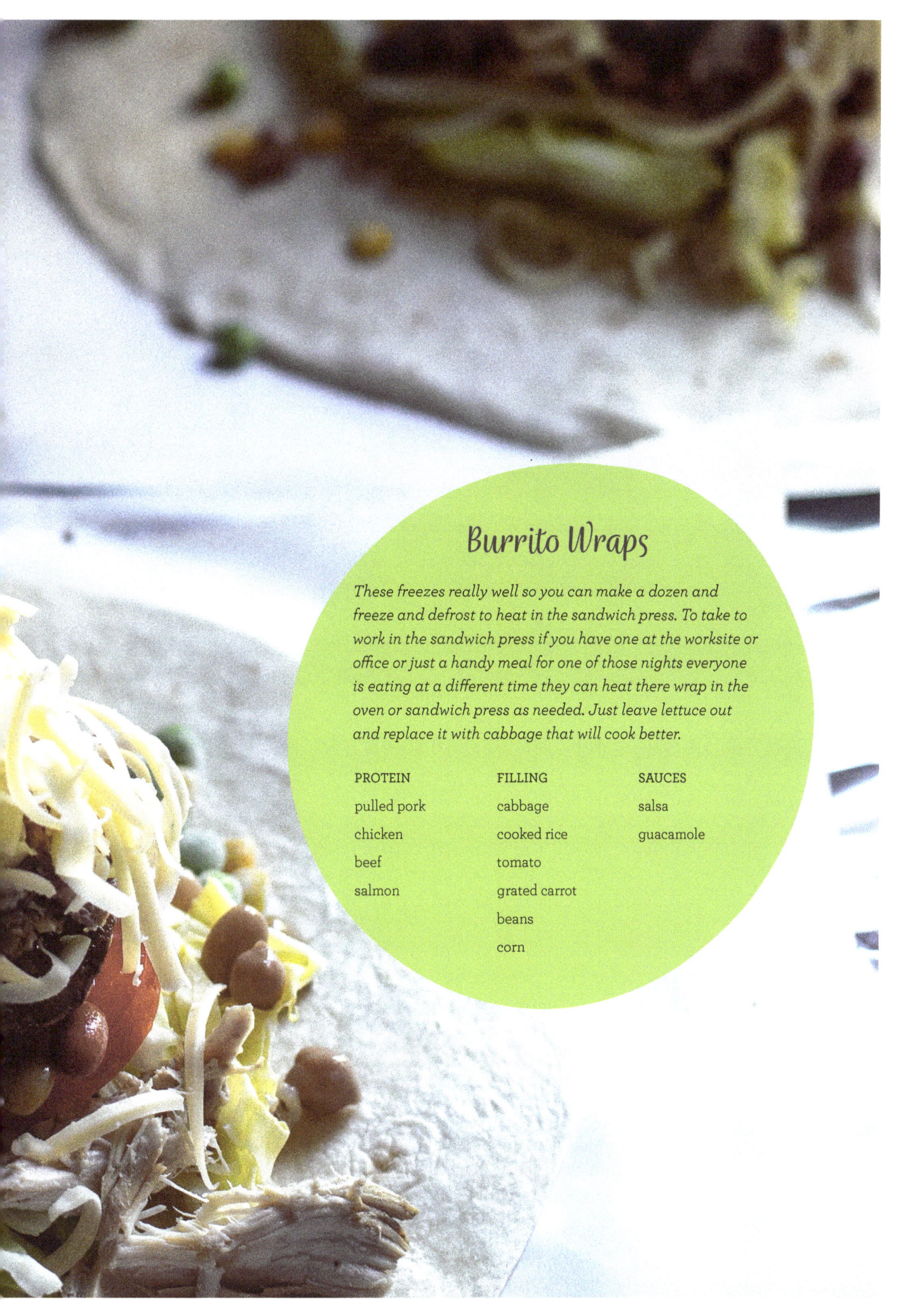

Burrito Wraps

These freezes really well so you can make a dozen and freeze and defrost to heat in the sandwich press. To take to work in the sandwich press if you have one at the worksite or office or just a handy meal for one of those nights everyone is eating at a different time they can heat there wrap in the oven or sandwich press as needed. Just leave lettuce out and replace it with cabbage that will cook better.

PROTEIN	FILLING	SAUCES
pulled pork	cabbage	salsa
chicken	cooked rice	guacamole
beef	tomato	
salmon	grated carrot	
	beans	
	corn	

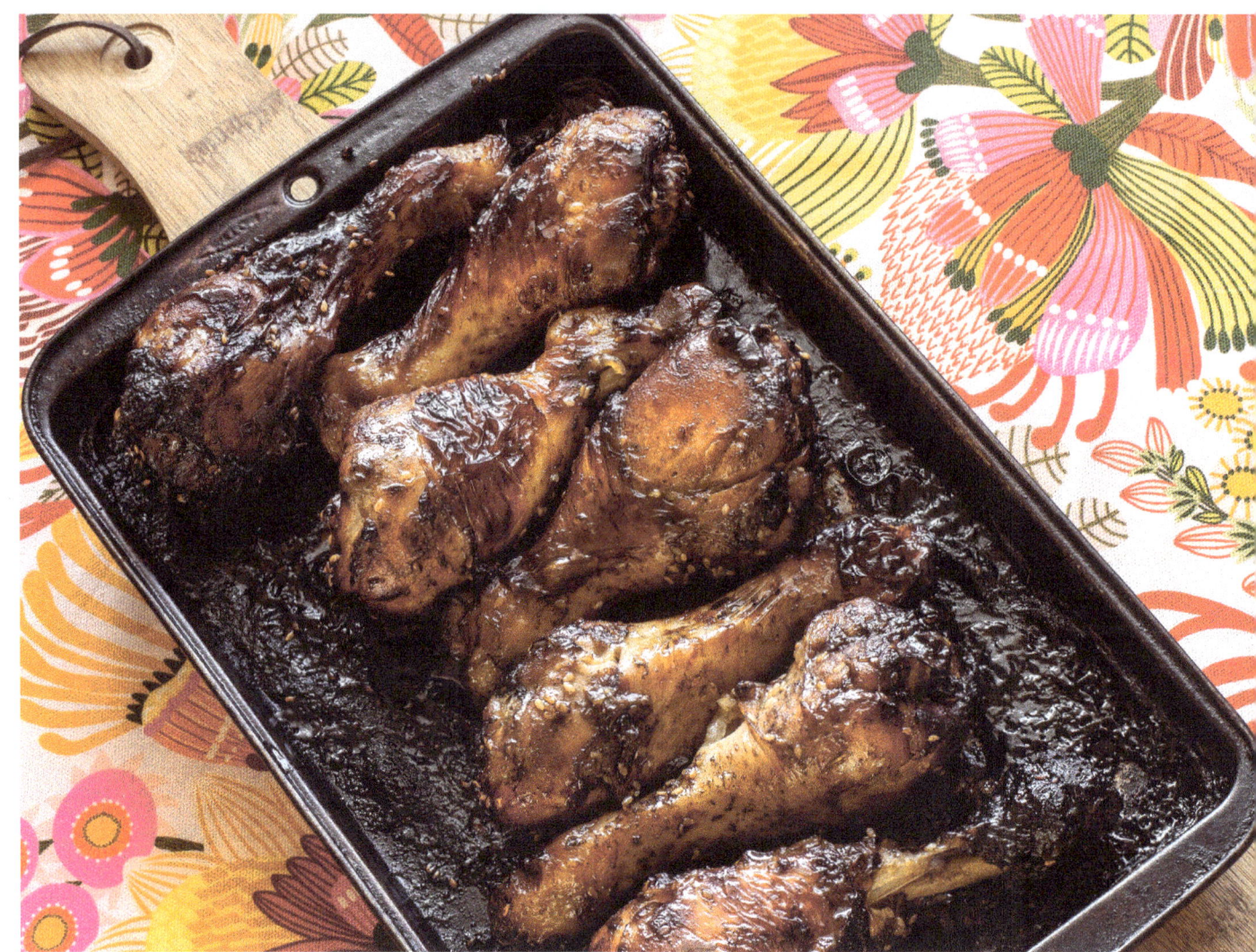

Baked Honey Soy Chicken Drumsticks

MAKES 12

You can use chicken thigh or breast on skewers to serve cold in the lunchbox.

12 drumsticks

2 tablespoons soy sauce

2 tablespoons honey

1 tablespoon extra virgin olive oil

2 cloves garlic

1 teaspoon Chinese 5 spice

2 tablespoons sesame seeds

Crush the garlic and mix with the soy, honey, oil, sesame and spices and coat the chicken well, leave to marinate overnight.

Heat the oven to 180°C.

Place the drumsticks in a baking tray on baking paper and bake the drumsticks for around 25 minutes or until cooked through.

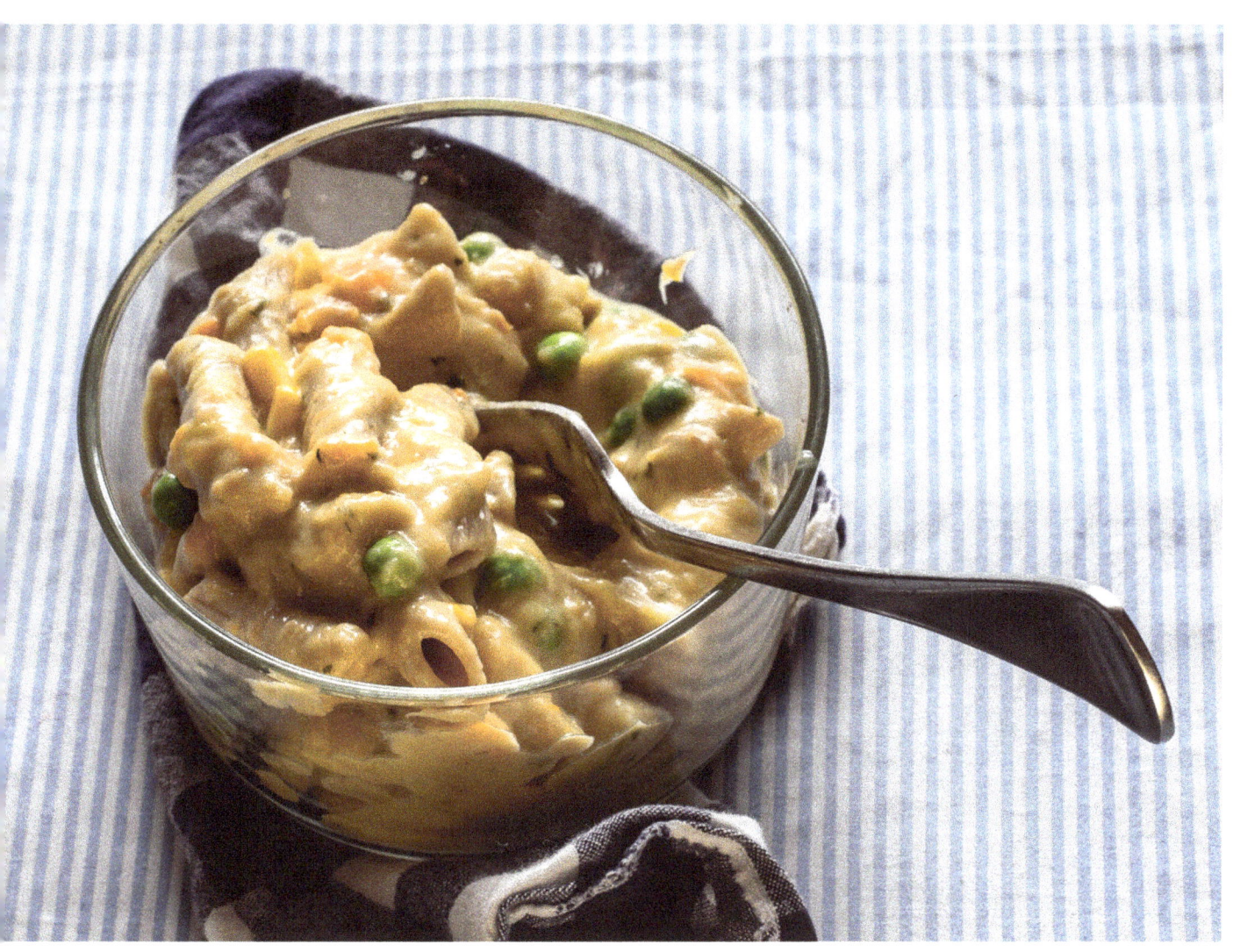

Tuna or Salmon Casserole

SERVES 4-6

25 grams butter

1 onion

2 cloves garlic

3 carrots

100 grams flour*

500ml milk

1 teaspoon ground fennel

1 tablespoon tarragon

1 tablespoon parsley

100 grams cheddar cheese

1 cup peas (fresh, frozen or tinned)

1 cup corn (fresh, frozen or tinned)

400 grams salmon or tuna (tinned, smoked or fresh)

2 cups cooked pasta

To make the casserole, melt the butter in a heavy-based frying pan over medium heat. Finely dice the onion, crush the garlic, add to the pan with the fennel and sauté.

Peel and finely dice the carrots, add to the pan and continue to sauté for 2 minutes. Add the flour* and cook for a further 2 minutes, stirring well to cook the flour.

Slowly add the milk whilst continuing to stir. Bring the mixture to the boil, reduce heat to a simmer, and stir until the sauce has thickened. This will take 5 to 10 minutes.

Finely chop the tarragon and parsley, grate the cheese and add to the sauce along with the peas, corn salmon and cooked pasta.

Scoop into warmed thermos.

*You can add 1-2 teaspoons of curry powder with the flour if you would like a different flavour

This can be pre-made placed into a casserole dish and then reheated in a 180°C oven for about 20 minutes to heat through.

Vegetarian Lasagne

SERVE 6-8

You will find my beef lasagne recipe in my first book 'The Real Food for Kids Cookbook' which is a family favourite, but I also love this vegetable version when I need a need a veggie meal. A great dish to make in summer when there are plenty of zucchini and tomatoes from the garden needing to be used up!

FILLING

1 large eggplant

2 large zucchinis

2 cups mushrooms

2 red capsicums

extra virgin olive oil

2 onions

4 cloves garlic

800 grams tomato

1 tablespoon basil

1 tablespoon oregano

PASTA

200 grams flour

2 eggs

CHEESE SAUCE

2 tablespoons butter

2 tablespoons plain flour

500ml milk

100 grams cheddar

50 grams fetta

50 grams parmesan

salt and pepper

Heat the oven to 180°C.

To make the pasta, put the flour into a large bowl and make a well in the middle. Add the eggs to the flour and combine. Turn out on to a clean surface or board and then knead well for at least 5 minutes until the pasta is smooth. Using a pasta machine set at number 1 (or at the widest opening setting) feed the dough through the pasta machine. Repeat this process 3 - 4 more times increasing the setting to a higher setting each time until the pasta is approximately 2mm thick and silky smooth.

To make the vegetable filling slice the eggplant into 1cm slices and rub salt into flesh and leave for around ½ hour, this will remove some bitterness. Rinse well and coat in oil and place on a baking tray. Slice zucchini coating in oil and place on a baking tray. Wash and slice mushrooms and coat in oil and place on the baking tray. Roast the zucchini, mushrooms and eggplant for around 15 minutes or until cooked through. Roast the capsicum by coating it in oil and placing in an oven tray and baking for around 15 minutes until the skin s crisp or burnt. Cool and peel of skin and discard seeds. Dice the onion and crush the garlic, then sauté them in a heavy based pan until the onion is soft. Add the crushed tomatoes, basil and oregano. Simmer for 20 minutes and then stir through all the roast vegetables that has been cut into a chunky 2cm dice.

To make the cheese sauce, melt the butter in a heavy based saucepan and add the flour and stir until combined. Add the milk gradually, stirring continuously until the sauce is thick and smooth. Add the cheese, stir through and season with salt and pepper.

In a lightly greased baking dish or tray, layer the vegetable filling and pasta sheets and top with the cheese sauce. Bake for 30 minutes until the top is golden brown and the lasagne is cooked through.

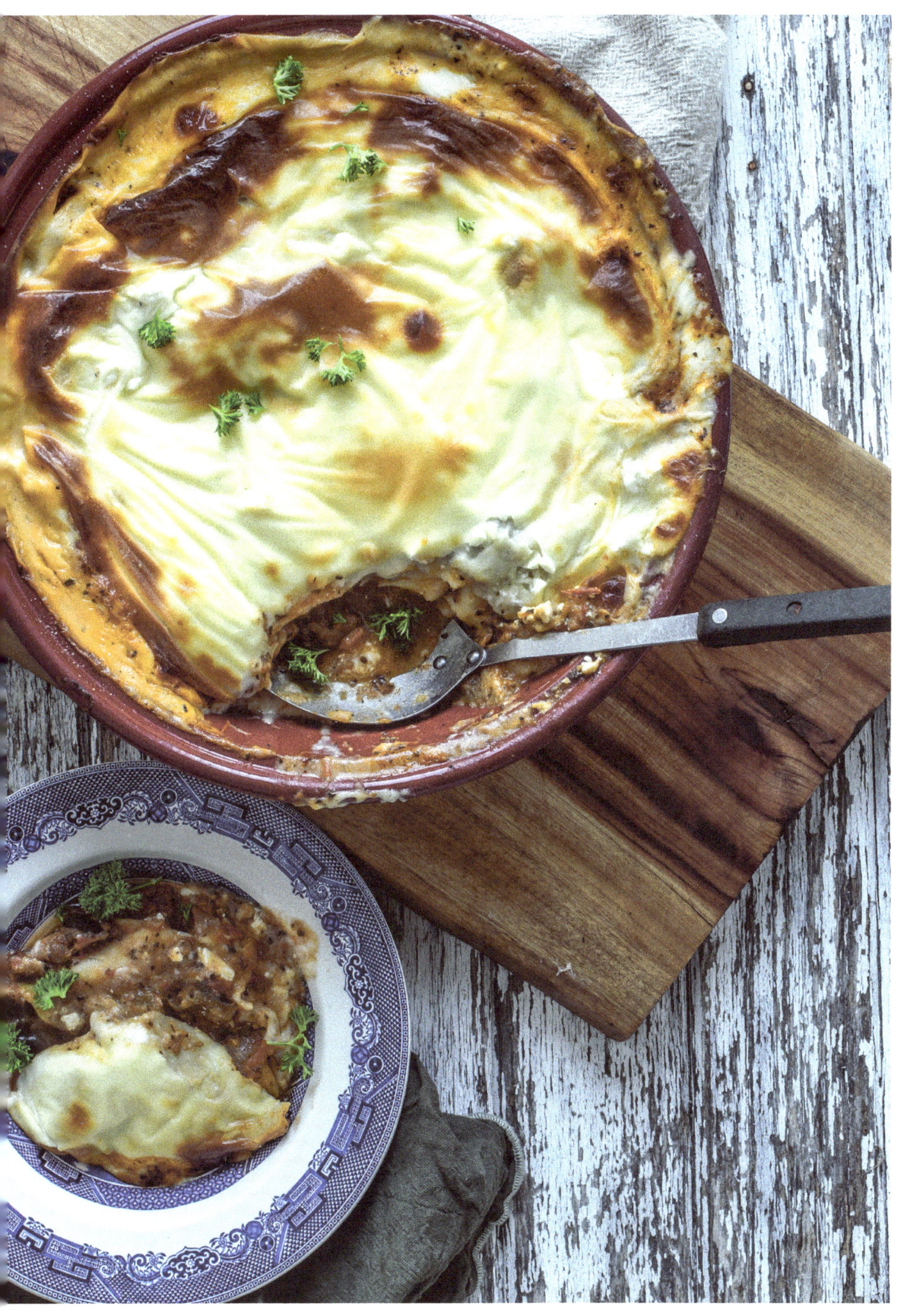

Loaded Baked Spuds

SERVES 4

Baked stuffed spuds are an easy and delicious lunch for the thermos at school or evening meal on the way home from activities. There are so many different filling ideas and when I was cooking school lunches there was rarely a child who did not like them. But they are not just for kids - with some leftover bolognaise, garlic butter, and coleslaw can be a nutritious and delicious dinner for the entire family too!

Depending on size of potatoes, 1-2 spuds per person

FILLING IDEAS

garlic butter, bacon and cheese

coleslaw

bolognaise and cheese

jalapeno peppers and mexican beans

pesto chicken and cheese

Heat the oven to 180°C.

Find large roasting spuds like Nicola and wash and prick with a fork and rub with extra virgin olive oil. Bake in a 180°C oven for around 30 minutes until cooked through and smash or cut in half. Load up with your favourite toppings.

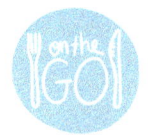 *Cook and chop up to serve in the thermos*

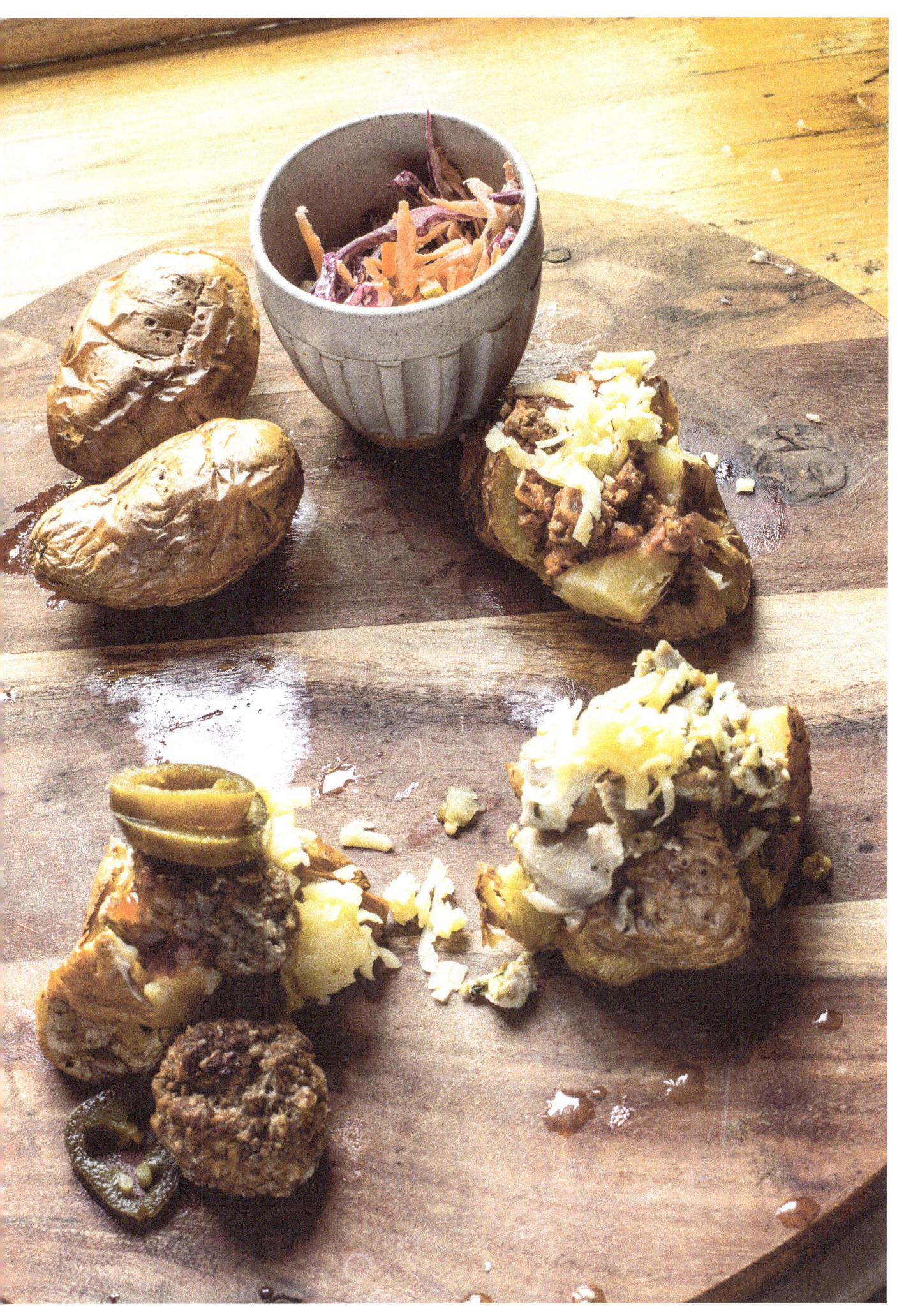

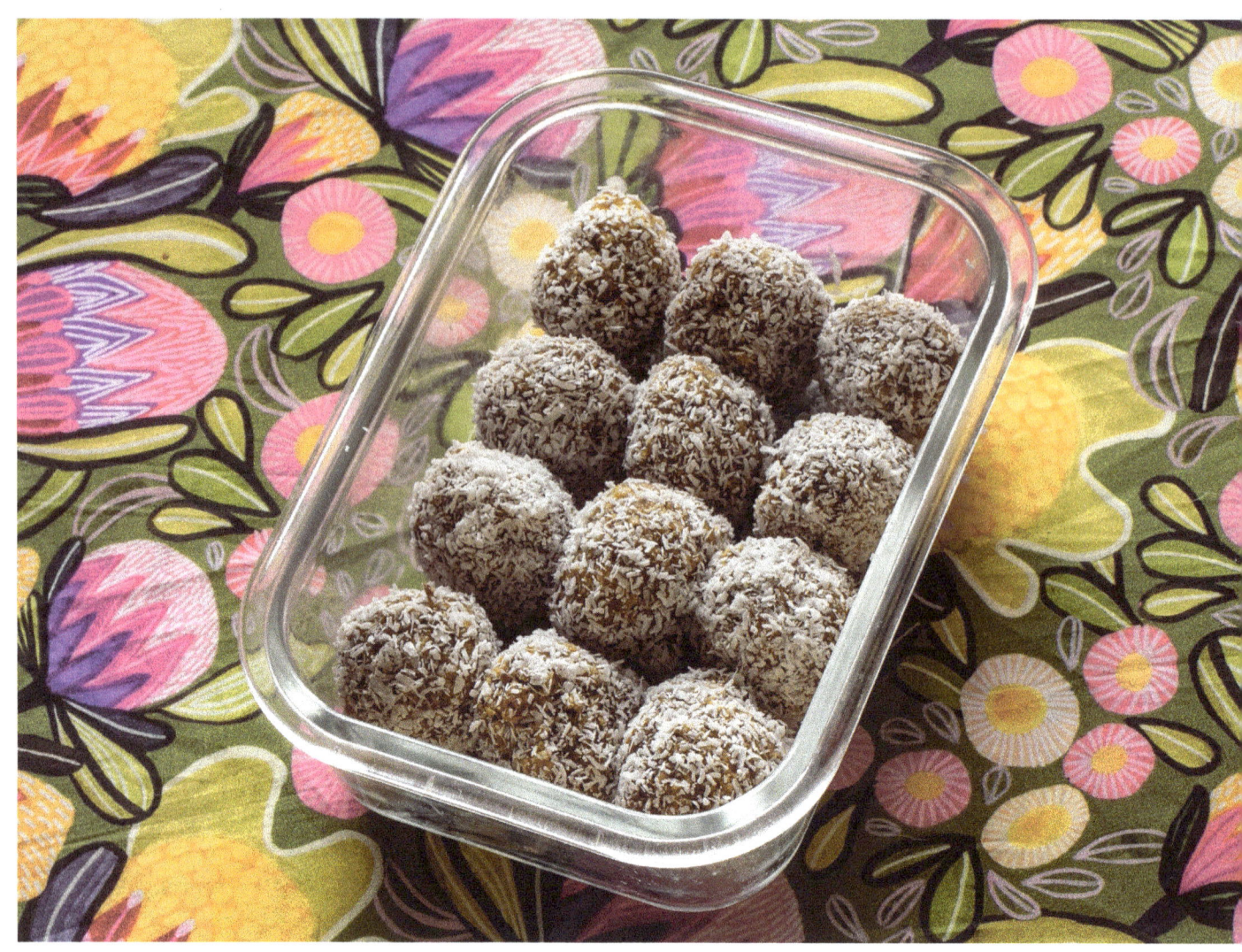

Apricot Bliss Balls or Slice

MAKES 20

You can use any combo of fruits and nuts, this recipe is nut free for the kids lunch box. You could use dates, vanilla essence, peanut butter, cacao lots of different ideas for flavours.

1 cup dried apricots

1 cup flax seeds

2 tablespoons honey

1 cup dates

1 cup dessicated coconut plus extra for rolling

pinch of cinnamon

1 ½ cup rolled oats

Place the ingredients in the food processor and blitz until smooth, roll each ball and roll in coconut. Store in air tight container in fridge for one week or freeze.

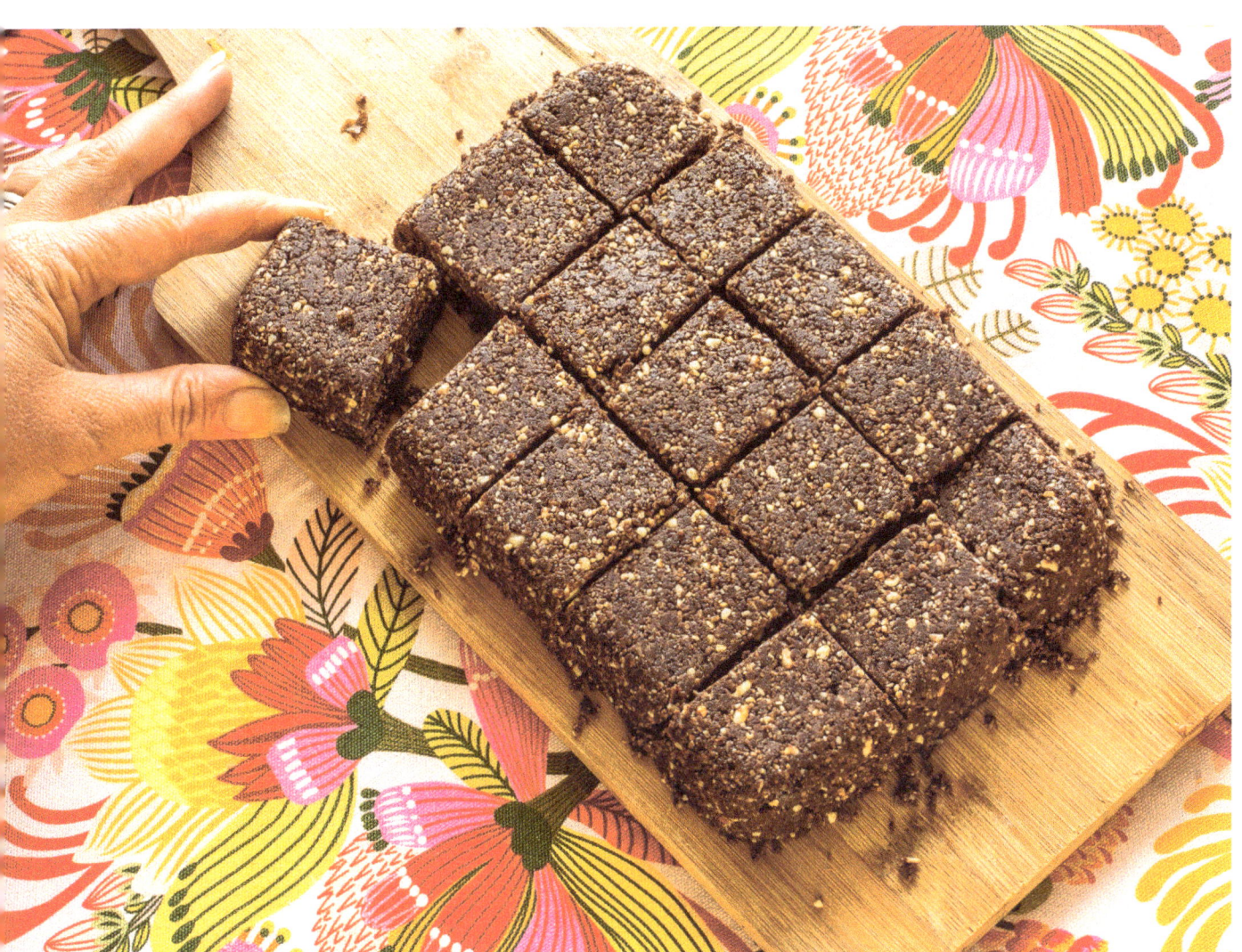

Chocolate Slice

MAKES 16

This is the EASIEST snack possible to make, and pretty healthy too, it satisfies my occasional sweet craving. You can use a mix of shredded coconut, dates, other dried fruits, nuts – almonds, cashews, cacao powder (or cocoa powder) you can roll them up into balls or press them into a tray for a slice. Use pumpkin or other seeds to replace the nuts, so they are nut free for the school lunchbox.

1 cup dates

1 cup dessicated coconut

1 cup cashews

¾ cup cacao powder

1 cup almonds

Put all ingredients into the thermocooker or blender with 1 tablespoon of water, blend for about 30 seconds and roll into balls or press in a tin to set in the fridge before slicing.

Fried Rice with Teriyaki Chicken

SERVES 4-6

Fried rice is an easy one to whip up for a quick meal in the thermos that the kids will eat. Add on top the teriyaki chicken (or use fish, salmon, pork or beef) for a decent serving of protein to make is a satiating meal. Use any veggies you need to use, other suggestions are broccoli, cauliflower, bok choy, celery

500 grams chicken

2 tablespoons soy sauce

2 tablespoons mirin (substitute with wine or white wine vinegar)

1 teaspoon honey

1 clove garlic

extra virgin olive oil for cooking

1 tablespoon sesame oil

3 spring onions

one rasher bacon

1 clove garlic

½ red capsicum

2 carrots

2 cups peas

⅔ cup long grain rice

1-2 tablespoons soy

Heat the oven to 180°C.

Cut the chicken into a 1cm strips. Crush the garlic and mix well with the soy, honey and mirin and coat the chicken well. To cook the chicken lay on a baking dish in one layer on a sheet of baking paper and bake for around 15 minutes or until cooked through.

Wash the rice and cook to the packet directions and cool. Chop the spring onion, bacon, capsicum, carrot into a ¾cm dice and crush the garlic. Heat a large heavy based pan over a medium heat and add oil, onion, bacon, carrot and garlic and saute until soft. Add the diced capsicum and rice and cook until heated through, add peas and heat through and season to your liking with soy.

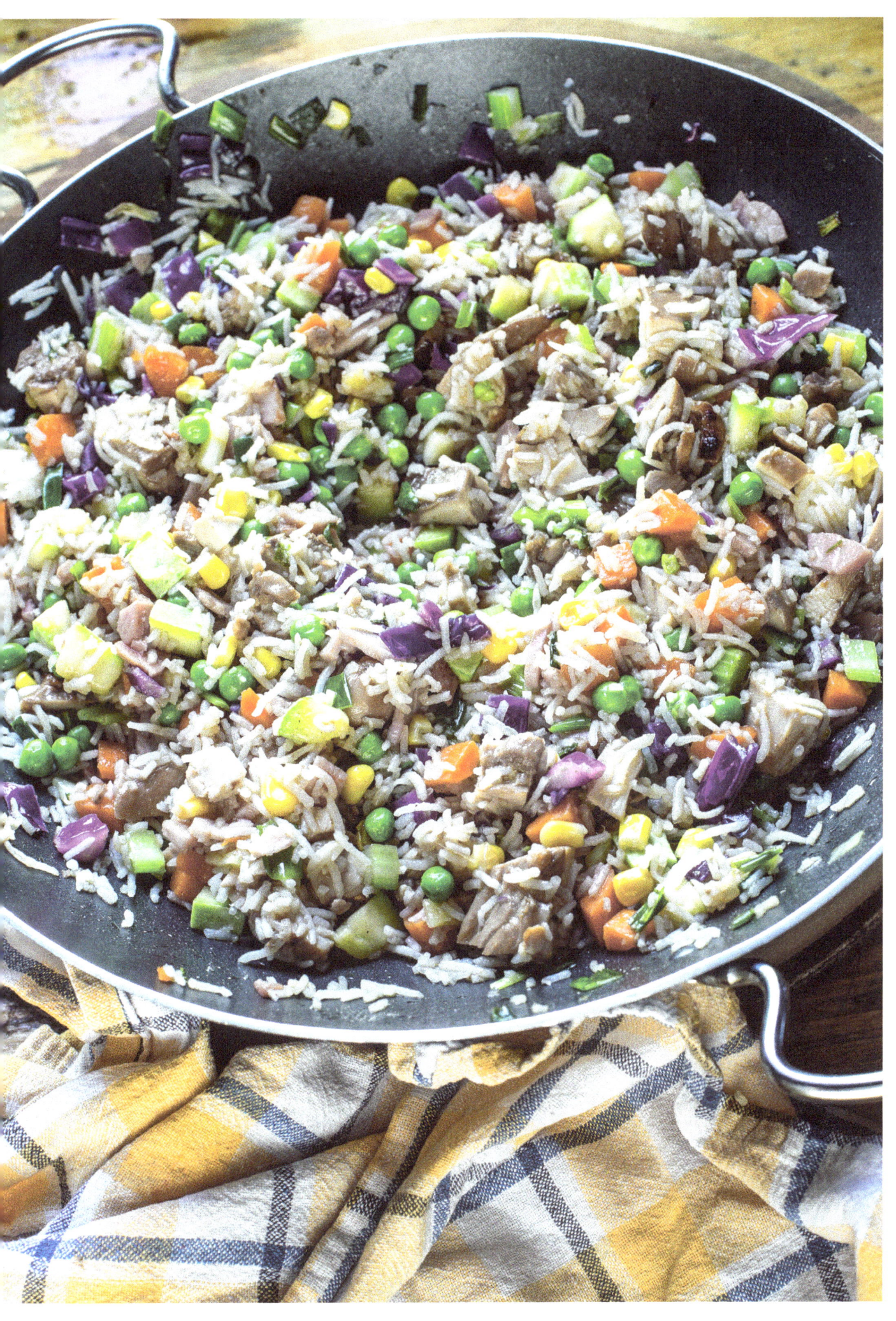

Burgers

SERVES 4-6

There is a beautiful and very popular fish burger recipe in my book 'Seafood Everyday' that has been extremely well received at different market stalls I have cooked at over the years and in homes. Or try a crumbed piece of fish or chicken for your burger. Swap the beef mince for pork, wallaby, lamb or a mix! We love packing a burger, egg, sliced cheese, wholemeal roll, lettuce, tomato and a coleslaw and then finding a council BBQ in a park to throw it all on a summers night, while waiting for one of the kids to finish activities. It never ceases to amaze me how bad a perfectly healthy meal can be destroyed so badly by big food companies who are only interested in profit. A home-made burger with all the trimmings and salad is a delicious satiating meal.

BEEF PATTY

500 grams beef mince

2 onions

2 tablespoons chutney

4 tablespoon fresh herbs like rosemary, thyme and parsley

4 cloves garlic

1 cup breadcrumbs

1 egg

extra virgin olive oil for cooking

TO SERVE

lettuce

beetroot

sliced cheese

chutney

wholemeal hamburger buns

tomato

grilled onion

fried egg

bacon

Crush the onion and garlic and finely chop the herbs and mix well with the mince, egg and breadcrumbs and shape into a burger patty.

Cook over a medium heat in a pan or the BBQ until cooked through.

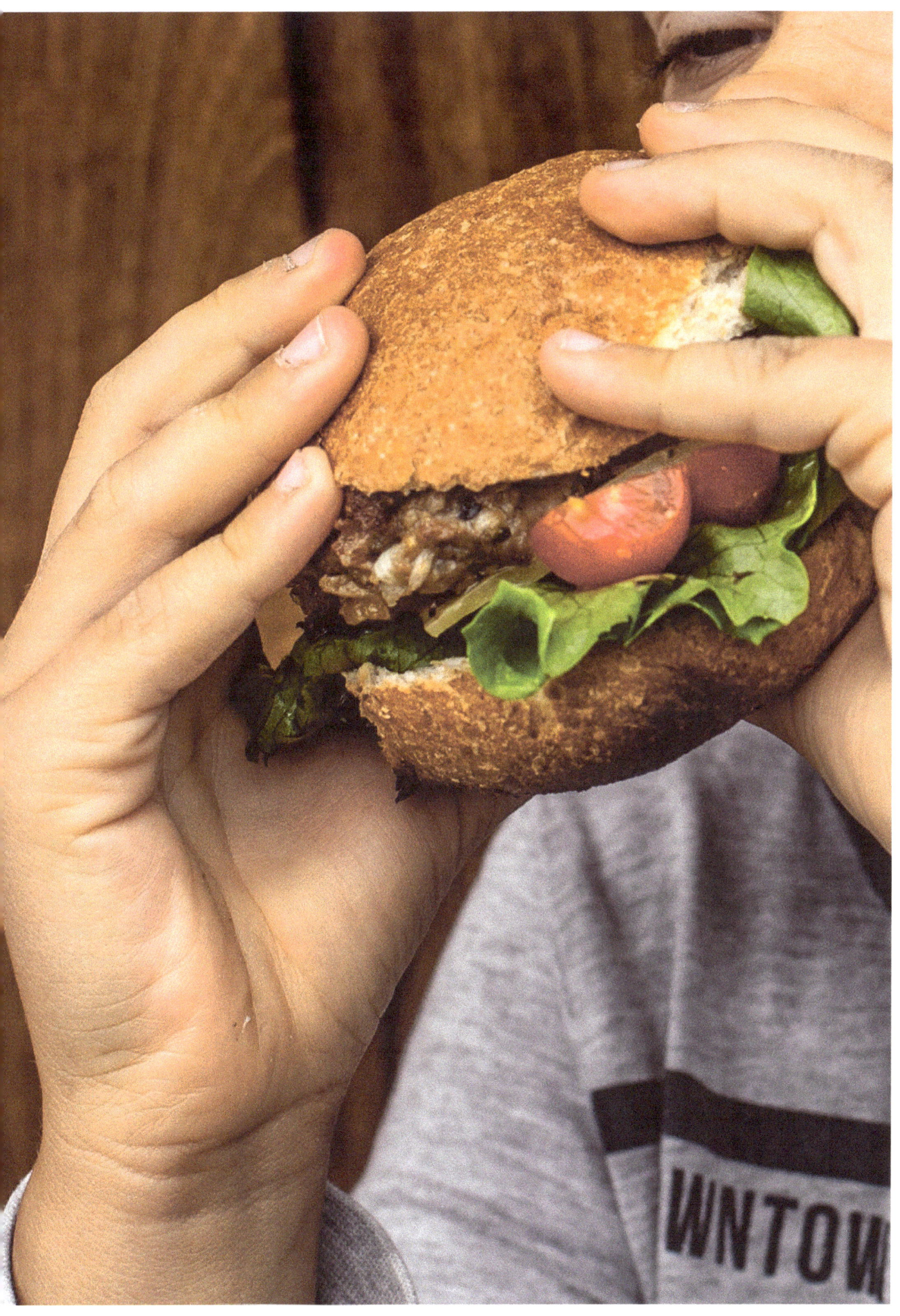

Fresh Vegged up Muesli

SERVES 4

There are 1000s of different combinations for this oat free "muesli". It is something we will enjoy regularly during the summer preserving season when there is an abundance of fresh fruit sitting on the bench ready to be bottled and we are consuming while fresh every way we can. Try and use fresh fruits with veggies like celery, cucumber, cauliflower or spinach mixed with any seed and nut. And it only takes a minute to whip up for an on the go breakfast or snack.

1 large carrot

200 grams cherries

2 apples

1 cup almonds

½ cup sunflower seeds

1 teaspoon cinnamon

½ teaspoon vanilla essence

TO SERVE

yoghurt

Put all the ingredients in the thermocooker or food processor and carefully chop into a rough chunky chop. Or grate or chop them. Serve with yogurt.

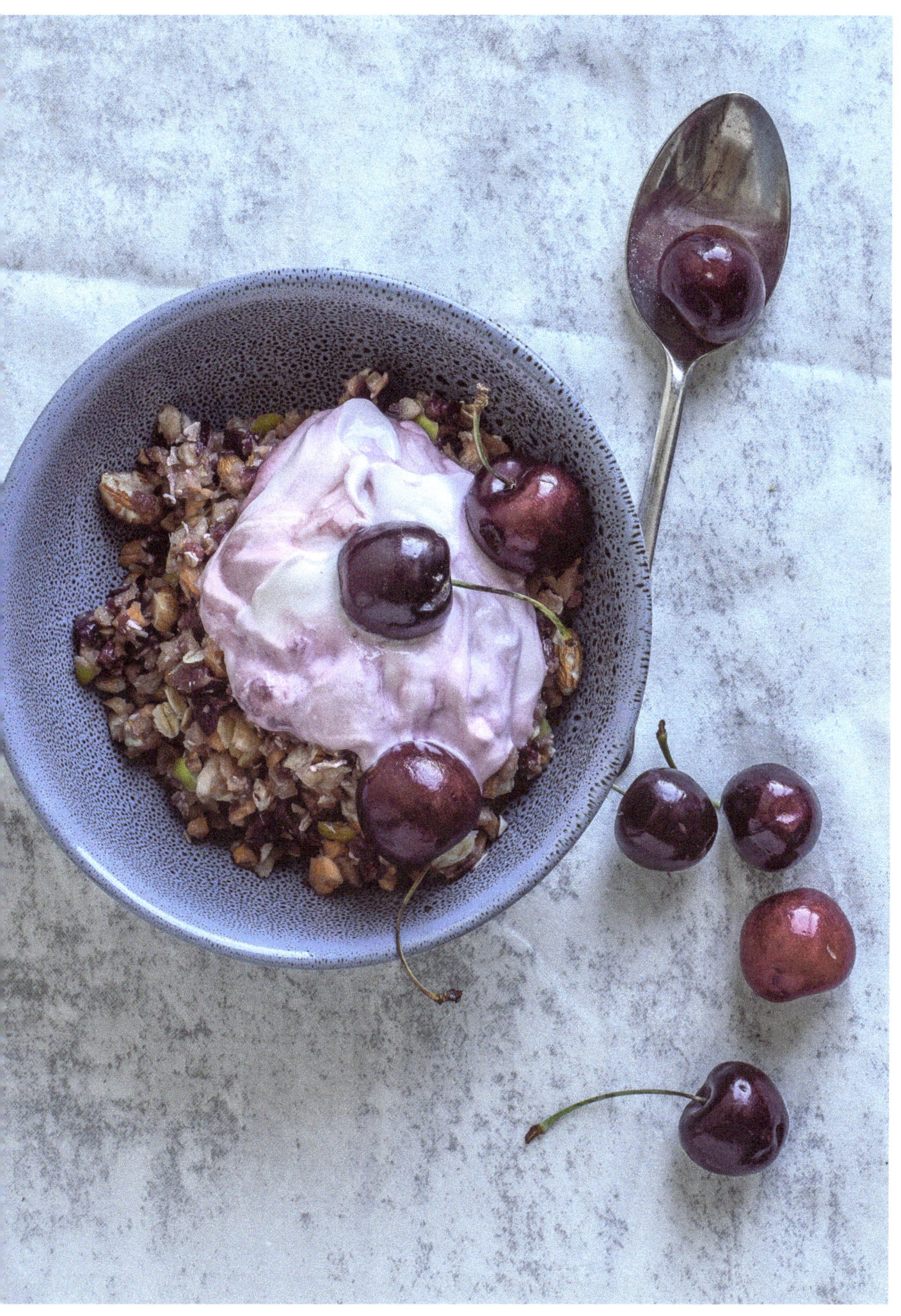

Occy and Broccoli, Bean Salad

SERVES 4

This bean salad made with solid veggies is a good one to have ready the day before a busy day. It can be made in advance and the flavours will only improve (with the leafy greens added just before eating). Not using too many tins is one habit I am trying to improve on for the waste factor, soaking and cooking the beans is better and more economical too but the tins in the pantry are handy for when you may be short of fresh veggies to whip this up.

200 grams cooked white beans

1 head broccoli

3 cloves garlic

½ small red onion

2 tablespoons basil

2 tablespoons parsley

sea salt

pepper

100 grams fetta

4 cups salad leaves

400 grams pickled octopus (see page 98)

Cut small florets of broccoli and bring a small pot of water to the boil. Blanch the broccoli for around 1 minute or 2 until just cooked. Drain and cool in ice water. Drain well.

Crush the garlic and finely chop the onion and mix will the broccoli, beans, chopped herbs, crumbled fetta and season with salad and pepper. Just before serving add the salad leaves and octopus.

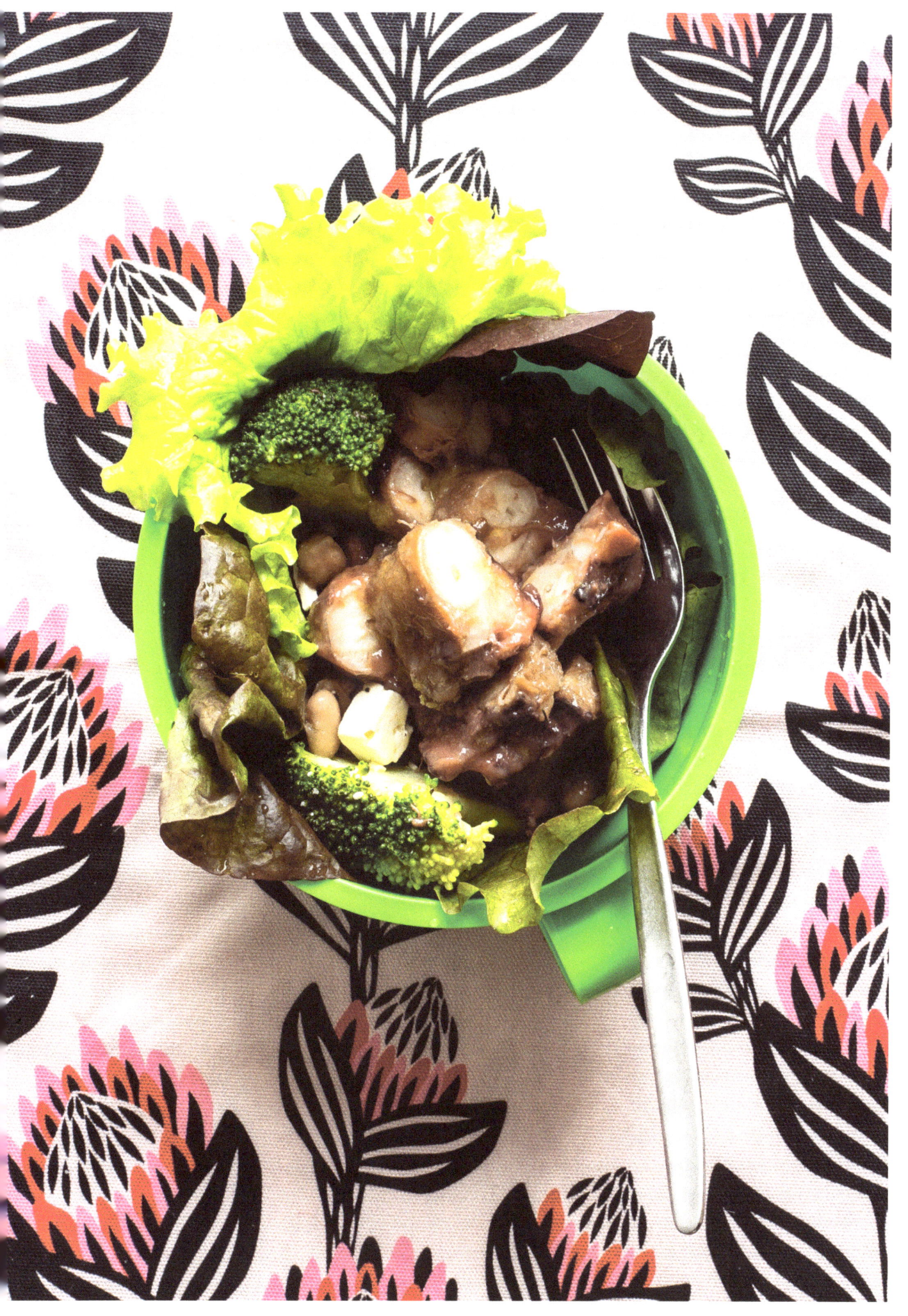

INDEX

A
Apple After School Muffins 84
Apple and Carrot Breakfast Muffins 36
Apricot and Almond Toasted Muesli 130
Apricot Bliss Balls 144
Apricot Chicken and Sage Buttered Cous Cous 124
Asian Flavoured Schnitzel Bowl 34

B
Baked Hazelnut, Pear, Berry and Cinnamon Porridge 131
Baked Honey Soy Chicken Drumsticks 138
Beetroot Salad 90
Berry, Apple Overnight Oats 135
Breakfast Trifle 134
Burgers 148
Burrito Wraps 136

C
Carrot and Pumpkin Soup 68
Cauliflower and Broccoli Mac and Cheese 32
Cauliflower Soup 69
Chicken, Brown Rice and Corn Soup 106
Chicken Ceaser 30
Chilli Con Carne 52
Chocolate Slice 145
Corn Salad 48
Cream of Broccoli and Bacon Soup 112

E
Egg and Bacon Pies 86

F
Fresh Vegged up Muesli 150
Fried Rice with Teriyaki Chicken 146
Fruit Leather 114

G
Garlic Pizza 25
Grilled Mediterranean Vegetable Panini 70
Green Chicken Curry 92

INDEX

Green Peppered Chicken Liver Pate 128
Guocamole 54

H

Honey Cinnamon Nut Bars 58
Honey, Lime Chicken 50
Honey and Mustard Slow Cooked Beef 116
Honey and Soy Chicken Nori Rolls 56
Honey, Soy Brown Rice Salad with Tassal Hot Smoked Salmon 122

I

Italian Chicken Meatballs 100

L

Lemon, Garlic and Herb Roasted Chicken 26
Lamb Kofta 76
Lamb, Lentil and Tomato Soup 110
Loaded Baked Spuds 142

M

Madras Beef or Lamb Curry 108
Mango Chicken 72
Mayonnaise/Aioli 25
Mediterranean Pasta Salad 44
Mexican Meatballs 94
Mexican Pulled Beef 42

N

Noodle Salad 88

O

Occy and Broccoli, Bean Salad 152

P

Pea Hummus 61
Pesto Mayo Chicken Salad 82
Pickled Octopus, Roast Pumpkin and Fetta 98
Potato and Bacon Salad 40
Pumpkin, Mushroom and Chicken Risotto 118

Q

Quinoa Roast Vegetable Salad 80

INDEX

R
Roast Beetroot and Fetta Salad 91
Roast Lamb 26
Roast Pumpkin, Spinach and Fetta Frittata 104

S
Salsa - Cooked 47
Salsa - Fresh 46
Savoury Rice Breakfast Porridge 64
Sichuan Pepper Pork Salad 96
Spiced Tassal Salmon 51
Slow Cooked Lamb, Silverbeet and Fetta Cannelloni 120
Slow Cooked Mediterranean Lamb Shoulder 62
Slow Cooker Roast Lamb and Cous Cous Salad 126
Smoothies 132
Spicy Breakfast Scones 102
Spicy Lamb Shank 78
Spicy Pulled Pork 74
Stock/Bone broth 28

T
Tatziki Dip 60
Thyme Polenta 116
Tropic Co Prawn, Broccoli, Apple salad with Honey and Mustard 38
Tuna or Salmon Casserole 139

V
Vegetarian Lasagne 140

W
Wraps 66

THANK YOU TO OUR GENEROUS SPONSORS

CAMPO DE FLORI

Discover a world of beauty at Campo de Flori. There's only one place in the world like Campo de Flori, where a whole world of beautiful tastes, views and experiences can be had in the one place. We are the only farm in Tasmania offering farm tours of saffron, lavender, olives with a cellar door for tasting and a ceramics studio where we can offer a true paddock to 'made here' plate on a farm.

Discover ceramics classes, take a farm visit, learn all about lavender, taste the beauty of the extra virgin olive oil and buy award winning saffron and culinary lavender from the farm gate. Located in beautiful Glen Huon, Campo de Flori is waiting for you to visit.

03 6266 6370
lisa@campodeflori.com.au
www.campodeflori.com

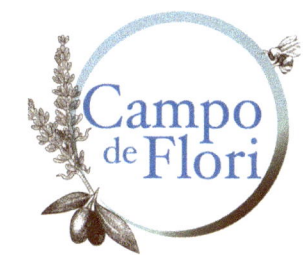

TASSAL

Our Home is Tasmania, a beautiful island with cool waters and a rich maritime history where our ambition to produce healthy, fresh Atlantic salmon began more than 30 years ago. From humble beginnings, we are Australia's largest producer of Tasmanian grown Atlantic salmon, our focus on quality and sustainability has underpinned our reputation as a global pioneer and leader. The management of food quality is of critical importance and we have extensive policies and procedures in place aimed at the consistent production of high quality, safe food for all consumers.

1800 652 027
www.tassal.com.au

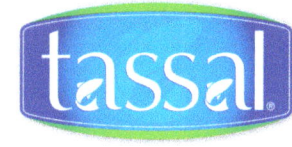

TROPIC CO

At Tropic Co, we are proud to provide high quality, world class tiger prawns with Australia's most sophisticated prawn farm network. Our farms are located across the coastline of Queensland and northern New South Wales with Australia's largest farm located near Gregory River.

Our farms, processing and supply chain is fully controlled and owned by Tassal Group, experts in aquaculture for over 35 years. We are excited to be delivering sustainable growth to the Australian Tiger prawn industry through innovation, technology and responsible farming, but our overarching strategy is to produce the BEST TIGER PRAWNS IN THE WORLD.

www.tropicco.com.au

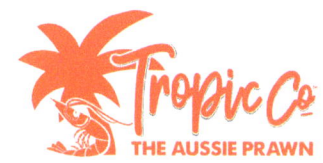

THANK YOU TO OUR GENEROUS SPONSORS

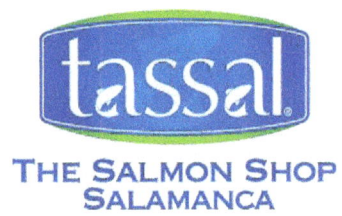

TASSAL SALMON SHOP

The Salmon Shop was created in 2007 as a centre to bring together everything that is Tassal salmon, giving us the opportunity to share our passion for salmon with the community. Located in a sea of galleries, theatres, cafés, craft shops and restaurants in Salamanca Square, the shop has quickly become a highly regarded fixture in this historic Hobart hub. More than just a shop, this must-experience destination includes a comprehensive range of delicious Tasmanian salmon products, deli stocked with delectable salmon accompaniments along with cook books and cooking utensils.

03 6244 9025
Tassal Salmon Shop, 2 Salamanca Square, Hobart Tasmania
www.shop.tassal.com.au

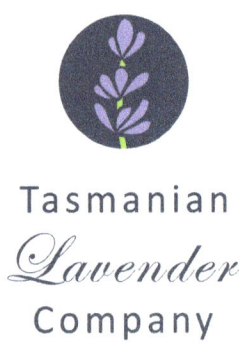

TASMANIAN LAVENDER COMPANY

Tasmanian Lavender Company represents a total transformation of our family farm business struggling through drought conditions and trying to find a way to remain viable. We set about planting our first 10,000 lavender plants creating a new way forward for the farm's future. In 2012 we decided to take a leap of faith and open our business up to the public. We purchased a property on the waterfront at Long Bay and planted a further 6,500 lavender plants. In 2014 after two years of planning and renovating, Port Arthur Lavender opened its doors.

Port Arthur Lavender's quality range of lavender products are displayed and available for purchase in an interactive visitor centre and café. We now hand make around 70 different products showcasing our lavender.

Port Arthur Lavender Farm
03 6250 3058
info@portarthurlavender.com.au
6555 Port Arthur Highway, Port Arthur Tasmania

Richmond Shop
03 6134 8100
info@tasmanianlavendercompany.com.au
25b Bridge Street, Richmond, Tasmania

YOUR BUSINESS

See your business advertised here? For information about sponsorship and advertising in future print runs of this book and new books visit www.eloiseemmett.com

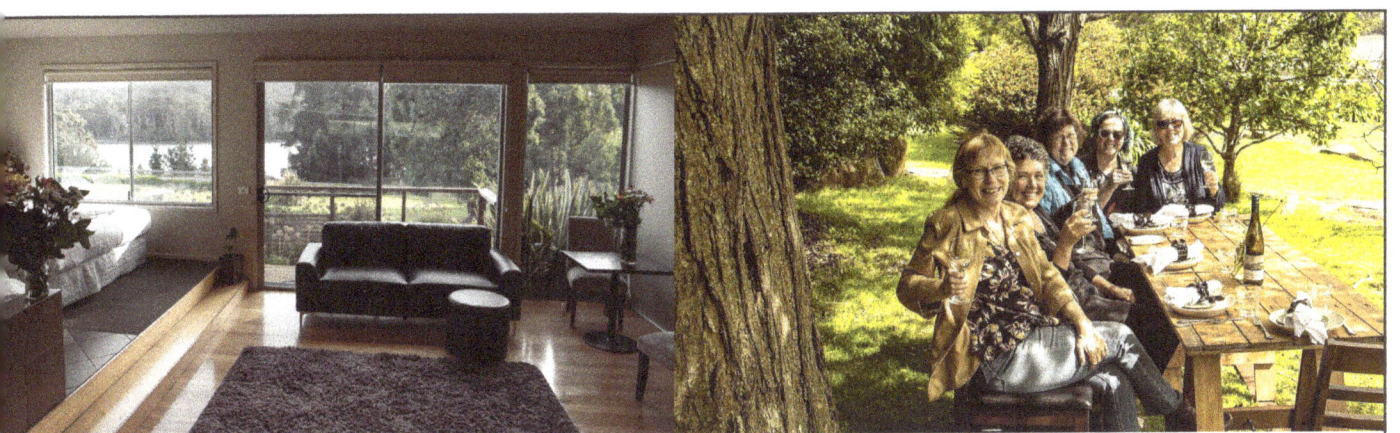

Little Norfolk Bay
EVENTS & CHALETS

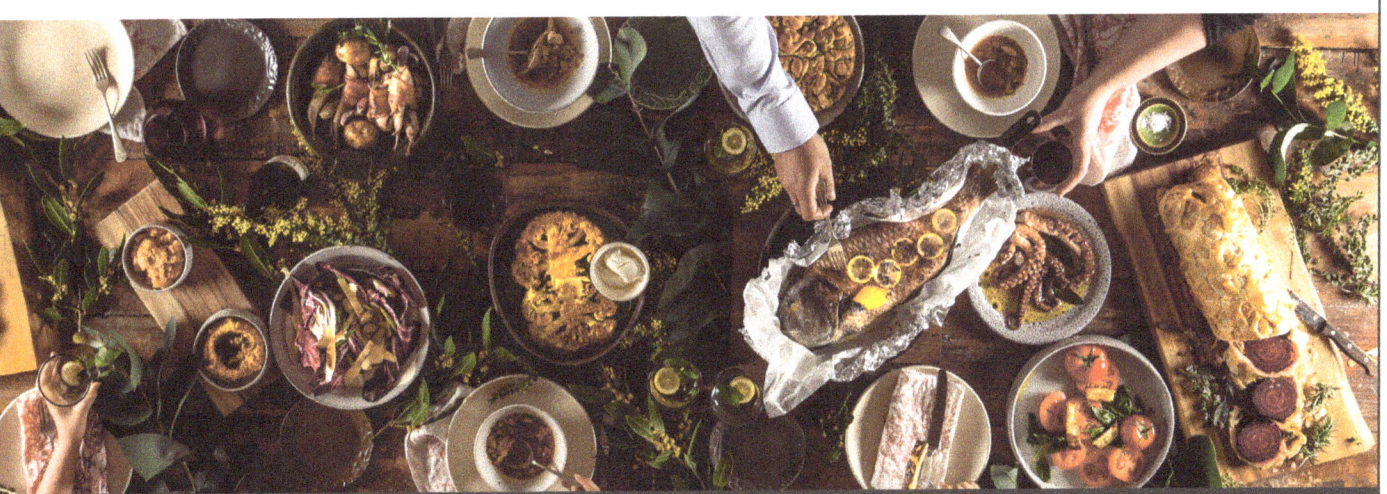

Accommodation, Cooking Retreats, Workshops and Indulgence Weekends in Taranna on the gorgeous Tasman Peninsula. Perfect for corporate or private gatherings and celebrations. Contact Chef and Host Eloise Emmett to design your unique experience.

www.eloiseemmett.com
www.littlenorfolkbayeventsandchalets.com

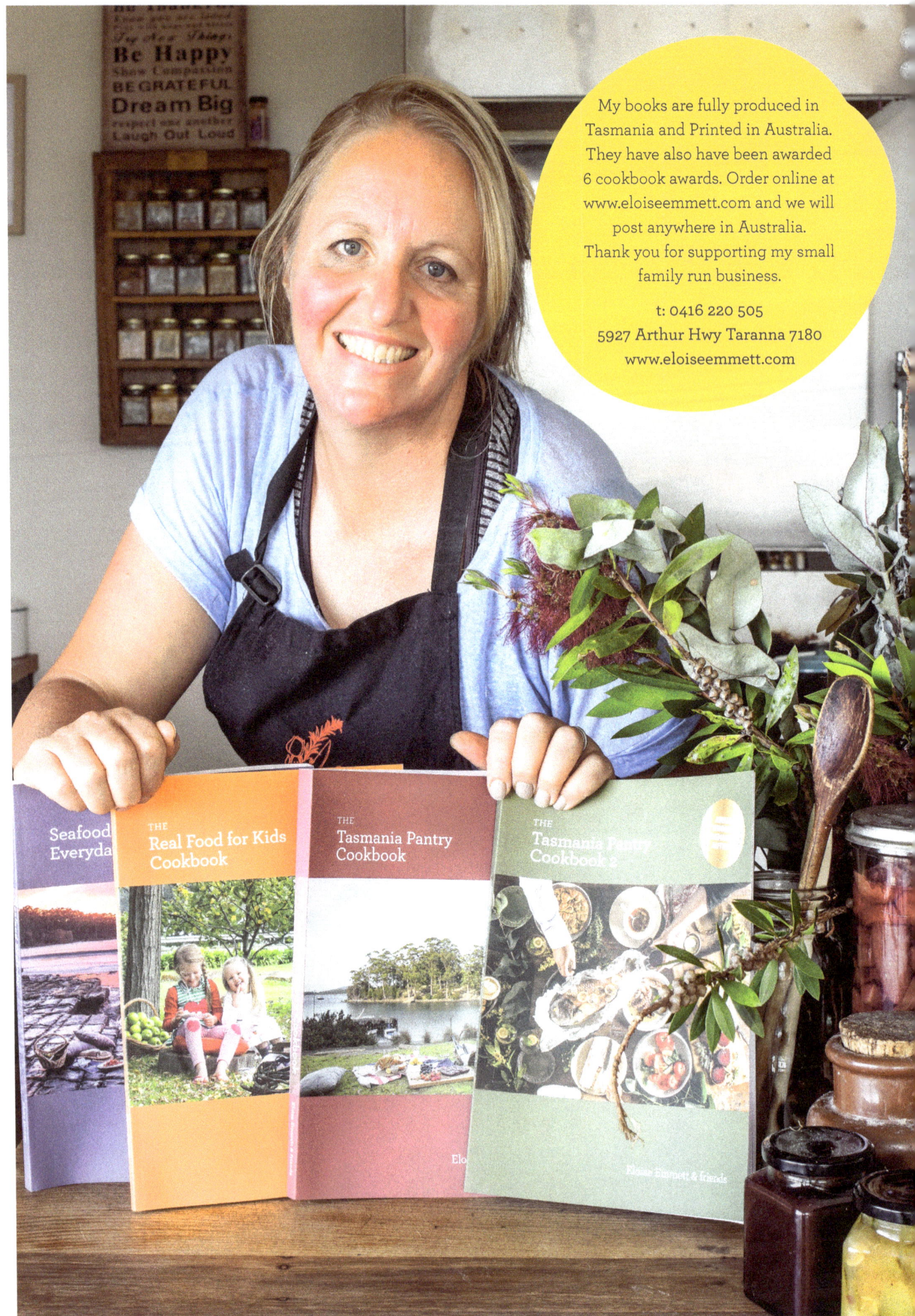

About the Author

Eloise Emmett is a Trade Qualified Chef with nearly 30 years experience in commercial kitchens, including 7 years as the Chef and owner of her own popular restaurant The Mussel Boys on the Tasman Peninsula. She now hosts weekend cooking retreats and indulgence weekends at Little Norfolk Bay Events and Chalets a luxury accommodation retreat and boutique cooking school.

Eloise has been writing and photographing recipes for her popular website eloiseemmett.com since 2012. In 2013 Eloise co-authored the *Bream Creek Farmers Market Cookbook*, in 2015 she published *The Real Food for Kids Cookbook* and in 2016 she published the multi award winning *Seafood Everyday*. *Seafood Everyday* won **Best Fish and Seafood Book in Australia**, and **Best Book by a Woman Chef in Australia**. It then went on to become the third best seafood cookbook in the world, when it and won third place in **The Best Fish and Seafood** category at the **Gourmand World Cookbook Awards**. In 2017 Eloise published the first print of *The Tasmania Pantry* and in 2020 she published the second edition, *The Tasmania Pantry 2*. Both books won national Gourmand Cookbook awards.

Eloise loves cooking, styling and photographing food and shopping for props at op-shops and markets. She has three children and with her fisherman husband and they live on the stunning Tasman Peninsula in Tasmania. Most of all Eloise loves educating families about how important cooking, preparing meals and eating real food. Her core message, is that cooking is not hard and is a lot more economical way to feed your family, and she encourages even the busiest families to prepare easy meals from real food.

www.eloiseemmett.com

Acknowledgments

Thanks for purchasing this book and supporting my small business. There are only two people involved in the production of this book, The designer Kylie, my bestie from Stokely 9 Design and The Art of Words Studio, and me. Unlike a published book that has a big budget and many staff involved. Although I have edited until my eyes go blurry about 200 times and I am not that great at sitting in front of a computer at the best of times, I am sure there will be the odd mistake or two. Let's hope they are little grammatical typos and not addition cups of chillies or something hideous like that! Please let me know if you see anything so I can fix for future print runs. Email me at eloiseemmett@gmail.com. Hopefully you can see them as little quirks in this handmade product, that is totally produced in Tasmania and printed in Australia!

Recipes, photography and words © Eloise Emmett

Design © Kylie Berry

No part of this book can be copied without permission, includes photocopying and photos of the pages.

Although I have researched the dietary information and other info carefully (for about 30 years!!) it is still only my opinion, so please always talk to a health professional. I will not be liable for any injuries or damage as a result of following the information and recipes in this book.

My four other books contain heaps of recipes that you will be able to pack up and eat on the go including lots of lunch box ideas. I have deliberately not included them so this book is full of all new recipes.

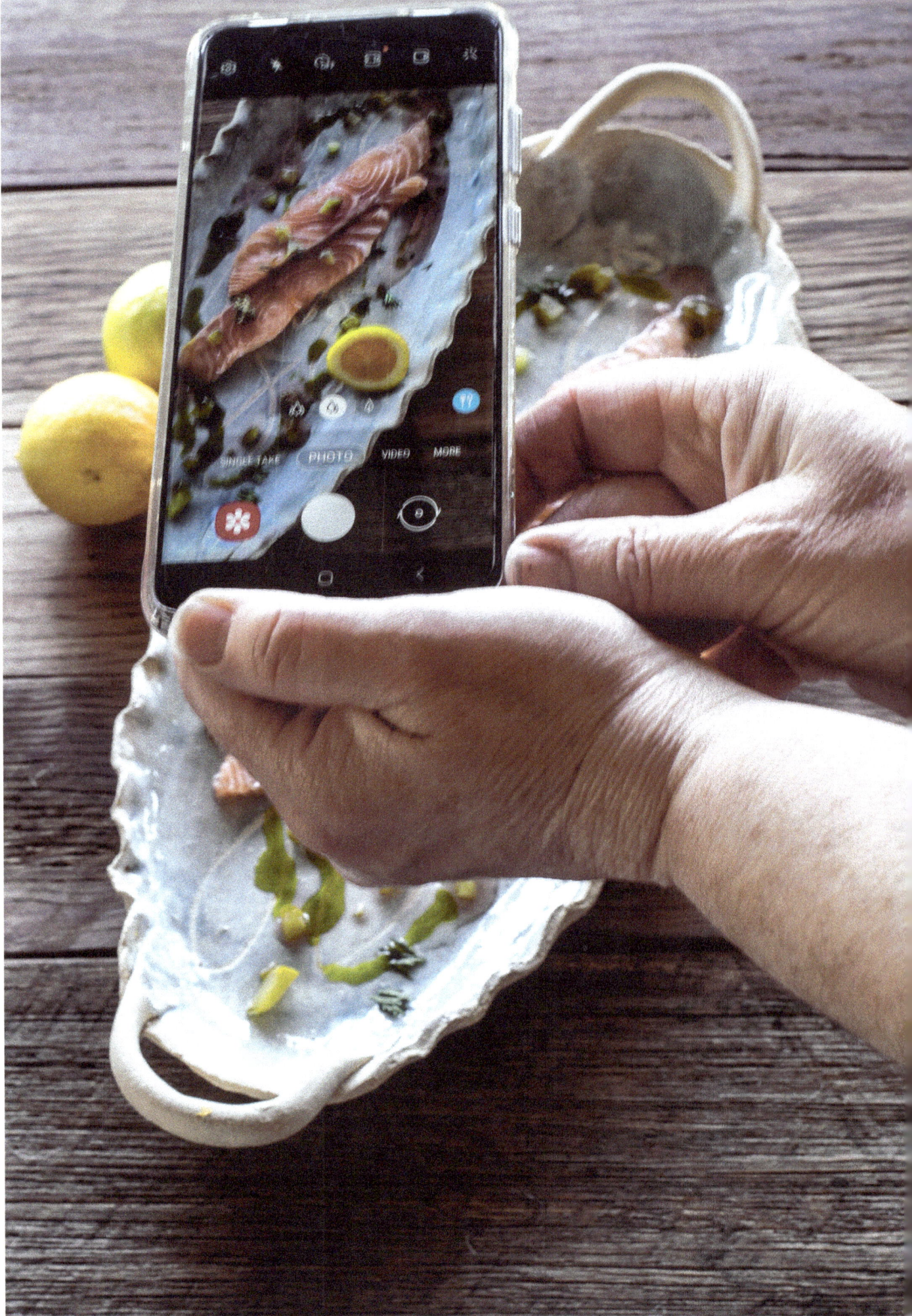

Feeling inspired?
Would you like to learn more?

You might enjoy my Workshops or Weekend Cooking Retreats at Little Norfolk Bay Events and Chalets!

I teach:

Seafood Cooking

Bread Making

Photography

Party Planning

Self Publishing

Phone Photography and Food Styling

Please find more information
at www.eloiseemmett.com

Eloise Emmett

CHEF   PHOTOGRAPHER   STYLIST

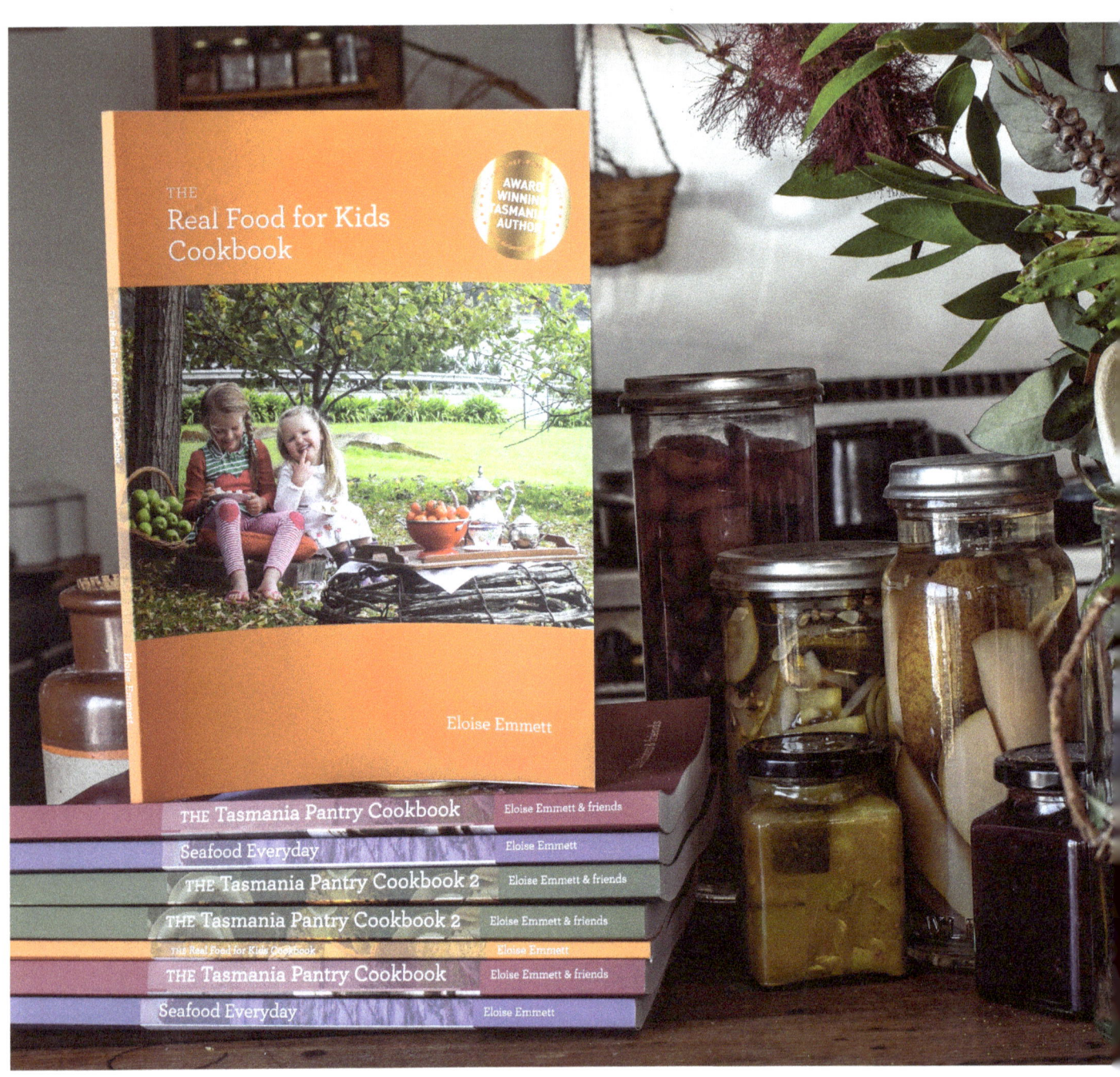

www.ingramcontent.com/pod-product-compliance
Lightning Source LLC
Chambersburg PA
CBHW040729020526
44107CB00086B/2993